Parachute Games
With DVD

SECOND EDITION

Todd Strong MS, MEd

Dale N. LeFevre, MA

HUMAN
KINETICS

Library of Congress Cataloging-in-Publication Data

Strong, Todd.
  Parachute games with DVD / Todd Strong, Dale N. LeFevre.— 2nd ed.
    p. cm.
  ISBN 0-7360-6363-3 (soft cover)
  1. Parachute games. 2. Physical education and training. I. LeFevre, Dale N. II. Title.
  GV1218.P34S77 2006
  793—dc22

                                        2005033372

ISBN-10: 0-7360-6363-3
ISBN-13: 978-0-7360-6363-0

The Web addresses cited in this text were current as of January 25, 2006, unless otherwise noted.

Acquisitions Editor: Bonnie Pettifor; **Developmental Editor:** Ragen E. Sanner; **Assistant Editor:** Carmel Sielicki; **Copyeditor:** Stephanie Ernst; **Proofreader:** Erin Cler; **Permission Manager:** Dalene Reeder; **Graphic Designer:** Nancy Rasmus; **Graphic Artist:** Dawn Sills; **Photo Manager:** Sarah Ritz; **Cover Designer:** Keith Blomberg; **Photographer (cover):** Ragen E. Sanner; **Photographer (interior):** Marion Crombie, unless otherwise noted. **Printer:** Versa Press

We thank Urbana Park District in Urbana, Illinois, for assistance in providing the location for the photo shoot for this book.

Printed in the United States of America   10 9 8 7 6 5 4 3

Human Kinetics
Web site: www.HumanKinetics.com

United States: Human Kinetics
P.O. Box 5076
Champaign, IL 61825-5076
800-747-4457
e-mail: humank@hkusa.com

Canada: Human Kinetics
475 Devonshire Road, Unit 100
Windsor, ON N8Y 2L5
800-465-7301 (in Canada only)
e-mail: orders@hkcanada.com

Europe: Human Kinetics
107 Bradford Road
Stanningley
Leeds LS28 6AT, United Kingdom
+44 (0)113 255 5665
e-mail: hk@hkeurope.com

Australia: Human Kinetics
57A Price Avenue
Lower Mitcham, South Australia 5062
08 8372 0999
e-mail: liaw@hkaustralia.com

New Zealand: Human Kinetics
Division of Sports Distributors NZ Ltd.
P.O. Box 300 226 Albany
North Shore City, Auckland
0064 9 448 1207
e-mail: info@humankinetics.co.nz

To Larry Diamond, who first taught us
to play with parachutes.

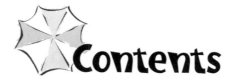

Contents

Part I Understanding Parachute Play

1 Discovering the Benefits of Parachute Play 3

Parachute Play Promotes Cooperation 4 • Everybody
Wins 5 • Parachutes Are Adaptable 5 • Parachute Play
Is Creative 6 • The Leader Can Play, Too 6 • Parachutes
Are Cost Effective 6 • Summary 7

2 Leading Parachute Games 9

Leading in the Spirit of Play 10 • Planning the Play
Session 11 • During the Play Session 13 • Ensuring
Safety 17 • Summary 19

3 Enhancing Developmental Skills 21

Social Skills 22 • Personal Behavior 26 • Perceptual
and Physical Skills 29 • Basic Motor Skills 32

4 Choosing and Caring for Your Parachute 37

Purchasing Your Parachute 38 • Distributors 41 •
Repairing Your Parachute 44 • Cleaning Your Parachute
44 • Decorating Your Parachute 45 • Storing and Caring
for Your Parachute 45 • Summary 46

Part II Learning the Games

5 Low-Activity Parachute Games 51

6 Moderate-Activity Parachute Games 83

7 High-Activity Parachute Games 121

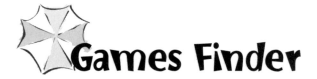

Games Finder

You want to play some parachute games, but with 59 games to choose from, you may feel overwhelmed. We appreciate that fact and therefore provide a games finder that will help you make your choices (see pages vii to viii). The secret is knowing what criteria are important for your particular play situation. Across the top row we have listed the criteria that we think are important, such as activity level (low, medium, or high) or when to play (beginning, middle, or end of the session). Scan across the top row to find the criteria that are important to you and then look down the games finder to find the characteristics you want. Look in the first column for the name of that game.

We suggest that you photocopy this finder so that you'll have it handy when you lead games. If you have other criteria that aren't listed here, you may want to design your own games finder.

As you lead and play the games and become more familiar with them, you may choose to eliminate the finder and just keep a list of games in your pocket. If you get stuck for a game in the middle of a game session, you can just pull out your list for a quick idea. That's what we do.

Name	Page number	Low, medium, or high level of activity	When to play	Included on DVD
Alligator	85	Medium	Middle	
Ball Surfing	87	Medium	Middle	
Big Bang	53	Low	Middle	●
Blow Up	54	Low	Middle	●
Cat and Mouse	123	High	Middle	●
Centipede	89	Medium	Middle	●
Circular Sit-Ups	91	Medium	Middle	●
Circular Tug	93	Medium	Middle	●
Climb the Mountain	95	Medium	Ending	●
Cop and Robber	97	Medium	Middle	●
Cover Up	55	Low	Middle	
Dodge 'Em	99	Medium	Middle	
Drag Race	56	Low	Ending	●
Floating Mushroom	57	Low	Middle	
Flying Parachute	125	High	Middle	
Free Play	59	Low	Beginning	●
Ghost Rider	100	Medium	Middle	●
Gophers	102	Medium	Middle	●
Group Balance	61	Low	Ending	●
Heartbeat	104	Medium	Beginning	●
Housekeeping	126	High	Middle	
I Dare Ya	127	High	Middle	
Igloo	62	Low	Middle	●
Interlocking Gears	63	Low	Middle	
It's in the Bag	105	Medium	Ending	●
Jell-O	129	High	Middle	●
Jellyfish Jaunt	130	High	Middle	
Jumbo Mushroom	65	Low	Beginning	●
Liftoff	107	Medium	Middle	
Merry-Go-Round	132	High	Middle	●

From *Parachute Games With DVD, Second Edition,* by Todd Strong and Dale N. LeFevre, 2006, Champaign, IL: Human Kinetics.

(continued)

(continued)

Name	Page number	Low, medium, or high level of activity	When to play	Included on DVD
Missile Launch	109	Medium	Middle	
Mushroom	66	Low	Beginning	◎
Ostrich	68	Low	Middle	◎
Over Under	69	Low	Middle	
Parachute Basketball	111	Medium	Middle	
Parachute Golf	70	Low	Middle	
Parachute Pass	71	Low	Ending	
Parachute Ride	72	Low	Ending	
Parachute Volleyball	112	Medium	Middle	
Pony Express	134	High	Middle	
Popcorn	136	High	Beginning	◎
Popovers	114	Medium	Middle	
Rabbit and Hound	74	Low	Middle	
Raceway	137	High	Middle	
Racing Heartbeat	138	High	Middle	◎
Rocking Chair	76	Low	Middle	◎
Sculpture	77	Low	Middle	
Shark	116	Medium	Middle	◎
Snake Tag	140	High	Middle	◎
Swooping Cloud	78	Low	Middle	
Top of the Pops	141	High	Middle	
Treasure Hunt	117	Medium	Middle	
Turnover	80	Low	Ending	◎
Wave Machine	118	Medium	Beginning	◎
Wave Rolling	142	High	Middle	
Wave Wall	81	Low	Middle	
Waves Overhead	119	Medium	Middle	
Who's Peeking?	82	Low	Middle	
World Record Merry-Go-Round	143	High	Middle	◎

From *Parachute Games With DVD, Second Edition,* by Todd Strong and Dale N. LeFevre, 2006, Champaign, IL: Human Kinetics.

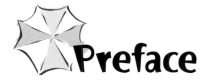# Preface

It's time once again to revive those underused parachutes bundled away in storage. If you're a teacher or recreation professional looking to enliven your group's physical activity program, *Parachute Games With DVD, Second Edition,* will inspire you to unpack that old parachute and bring it back to life. If you've never played with parachutes, you'll want to buy one today and introduce this exciting new activity to your players.

Whether you're a novice or you're already a parachute games aficionado, *Parachute Games With DVD, Second Edition,* will

- add to the number of games you already know,
- give you ways to categorize games for different play groups and settings,
- provide advice on how to present the games,
- group games by developmental skill, and
- show you how to care for and maintain your parachute.

The idea for this book came while its authors were watching a group of elementary school children play with a parachute during their physical education class. Watching the kids and teachers having so much fun reminded us of all the great parachute games and activities we have learned, played, and shared. So, we decided to put our experience and enthusiasm into a book, this time utilizing a helpful DVD to guide you through some of the activities. *Parachute Games With DVD* is our way of sharing our excitement with you. Updates to this second edition include clarification to some game descriptions to make them even easier to understand. Photographs demonstrate how the games are played, as well as convey the fun that your players will experience. With the DVD that is now included, you can see for yourself how to lead the games and how the players interact with each other, the equipment, and the play leader. Look for the DVD icon shown here to signal a lesson found on the DVD.

This book is divided into two parts. In part I we include everything you need to make parachute games exciting, instructional, and safe in a variety of settings. In chapter 1 we look at the benefits of parachute play and suggest low-cost items that can complement your activities. In chapter 2 you'll find useful tips on how to lead the games so that you can add to the playfulness, even while you explain the rules. We'll help you become aware of different play leadership styles and techniques and show you the best way to present the games.

Chapter 3 lists games by the skills needed to play them, in recognition of the close association between the enhancement of developmental skills and the learning process. To ensure that you get full value from the equipment, chapter 4 identifies features to look for when you buy a parachute, including a list of sources. We also recommend the best ways to store your parachute and give tips on how to maintain and mend it so that it will last. Since publication of the first edition of *Parachute Games,* the popularity of using parachutes as a fantastic piece of equipment for group games and recreation activities has continued to rise. Although the basic shape of a play parachute hasn't changed, new chutes are available in new designs. To reflect these new options, we have updated chapter 4, "Choosing and Caring for Your Parachute," to provide you with the most recent information on purchasing and maintaining your play chute.

In part II you'll find a comprehensive list of our favorite parachute games. We bring these games to life, using photographs to illustrate our explanations and descriptions. We precede chapter 5 with three sample play-sessions to pique players' interest. Then we divide the games into categories—low activity in chapter 5, moderate activity in chapter 6, and high activity in chapter 7—and present them in alphabetical order. A handy games finder helps you quickly identify which games will fit your immediate needs.

The format in which each game is presented in chapters 5 through 7 will help you figure out your personal list of great parachute games. We share tips on what games work well in specific settings, such as the type of surface on which the parachute will be used. We consider the age, size, number, and diversity of the players, plus factors such as intensity level of the game, to help you choose appropriate games. Finally, we suggest interesting sequences of games that work well together to help you design a fun, meaningful play session no matter where or with whom you are playing.

Along with the DVD, the two most exciting and important changes to this revised edition of *Parachute Games With DVD* are the two new categories: Variations and Teaching Tips.

• Variations is our way to fit even more great parachute games into this book without making the book more expensive. Imagine discovering a great game and then finding that—with a few simple changes—this great game morphs into a second great game. That's the purpose of Variations. It effectively doubles the number of games in the book. We don't recommend that you play all of the variations of a game one after the other or even during the same play session. Instead, try out a new variation of an old game during a different play session. These variations will help maintain your parachute play as a fun, fresh activity.

• Teaching Tips is our way of sharing the experience and insights we have gained from our years of leading and playing parachute games with all sorts of different people, in all sorts of different settings. In these tips we point out strategies that have helped optimize our play sessions.

Many of the games were learned from fellow play leaders and players. If you know of and would like to share a great parachute game, activity, or variation that is not covered in this book, please send your idea to Todd Strong; P.O. Box 204; Point Roberts, WA 98281; USA. Of course we will be happy to credit you and your organization for the idea in a future edition.

We hope that sharing our experience and enthusiasm in this book allows more and more people to play. Please enjoy, and have as much fun using this book as we had in researching and writing it.

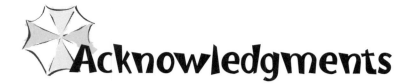

Acknowledgments

Thank you to all the friends, family, and others who participated in the photo sessions. Particularly, thank you to the Mendocino Elementary School (CA); Fort Bragg Middle School (CA); East Oxford First School (UK); East Oxford Woodcraft Folk (UK); Cardinal Newman Middle School (UK); and Playschemes at Blackbird Leys, Temple Cowley, and Rosehill (UK).

Thank you to the day campers and staff of the Urbana Park District (IL) who participated in the DVD and photo session.

Thanks also to the wonderful folks at Human Kinetics. Their kindness, passion, and attention to detail are much appreciated. In particular, thanks to Ragen Sanner, Carmel Sielicki, Lori Cooper, and Bonnie Pettifor for all of the many ways they helped to improve the book.

Part I

Understanding Parachute Play

The word *parachute* comes from the Latin root *para*, which has evolved to mean "to protect," and from the French *chute,* meaning "fall," and roughly translates as "protecting from a fall." Although Leonardo da Vinci had already sketched an early parachute model by 1495, it was not until the late 18th century that people began using parachutes to drop safely from the sky. Jean Blanchard, a noted balloonist of the period, amused audiences by dropping animals attached to parachutes from his airborne balloon. Andre Garnerin was a bit braver: On October 22, 1797, he cut himself from a balloon and safely descended some 3,000 feet (914.4 meters) to the ground in the first successful parachute drop involving a human. Polish aviator Jodaki Kuparaento was the first to use a parachute as an emergency lifesaving device on July 24, 1808, when he jumped from a balloon that was on fire. Since that first jump to safety, parachutes have saved thousands of lives.

As parachute designs improved, the new sport of skydiving became more popular. By 1936, skydivers were competing with one another, jumping out of planes and flying freely for thousands of feet before opening their parachutes. Thanks to improved designs, parachutists now have maneuverability and accuracy that were unthinkable in the sport's early days.

Whoever first thought of using a parachute as a giant game apparatus remains unknown. When relatively inexpensive used parachutes appeared in army-surplus stores in the 1960s, playful pioneers found the opportunity and inspiration to create new recreational and physical education activities. Larry Diamond, in particular, amazed us in the 1970s with his giant parachute wizardry at New Games festivals in the San Francisco Bay area.

Today parachute makers design and build colorful play equipment specifically for people to enjoy together on the ground—and we hope you will use *Parachute Games With DVD, Second Edition* to do just that.

Discovering the Benefits of Parachute Play

1

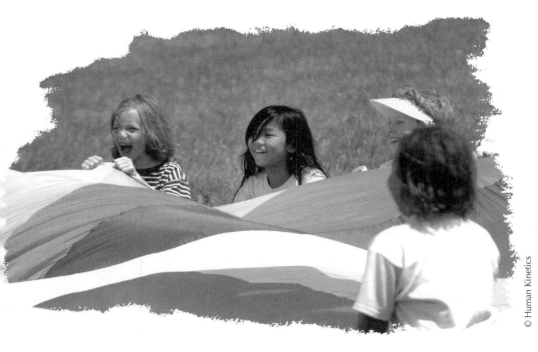

When the first daredevils used parachutes to float safely down to earth, they probably had no idea of the advances that were to come. Today's parachutes allow for control that was unheard of in the beginning days of skydiving. Those early parachute jumpers also could not have imagined how much fun a group of people could have playing with a parachute while remaining earthbound. This chapter presents some of the benefits of playing with a parachute.

Parachute Play Promotes Cooperation

Playing with a parachute promotes teamwork and cooperation. When playing with a parachute, everyone shares the same piece of equipment at the same time. In sports such as football, basketball, or volleyball, the players use the same piece of equipment (i.e., a ball), but rather than share it, they compete to control it. In parachute play, instead of fighting to determine who manipulates the equipment, all the players are in contact with the parachute, and they work together toward a creative end. Even when teams do compete against each other, as in the game of Popovers, people still share the parachute. This shared control gives a more cooperative feel to the game than if people were always fighting over control of the equipment.

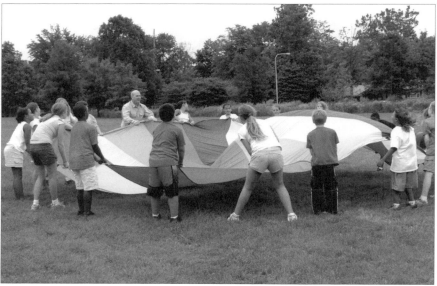

©Human Kinetics

Teamwork and cooperation are integral skills when playing with a parachute.

Because play parachutes are round, the players naturally form a circle around the edge. Being in a circle lets all the players see each other, and this visual contact creates a group awareness that promotes more cooperative and safer play.

In contrast, imagine the same group of people playing with an Earthball. An Earthball is an inflated ball 6 feet (1.8 meters) in diameter, painted to look like the Earth. In most Earthball games each player focuses on the ball rather than on the other players. An Earthball is so big that players on opposite sides often cannot see each other. The excitement of playing with such a large ball combined with the absence of awareness of other players means that, without supervision, people could get run over. Parachutes share the same bigger-than-life quality of an Earthball but are inherently safer. The circular formation around a parachute forces people to be aware of and cooperate with the group.

Everybody Wins

There are no losers in parachute games. Many parachute games don't even involve competition. Parachute activities often consist of everyone playing together to achieve a shared goal. Some of the games, however, are competitive. Many of these competitive games involve the entire group playing together on the same team, with the team competing against itself. For example, the World Record Merry-Go-Round game involves competition, but the team is trying to beat its own previous record.

Even in games that involve competition between different teams, the focus is on playing, not on winning. Each round lasts for only a short time, and there is no stopping between rounds to award points or hand out medals. The players are having so much fun that they want to get on to the next round or the next game. No one worries about winning or losing.

Parachutes Are Adaptable

Parachute games are flexible. You can play with a parachute for five minutes or for an hour. Because parachutes are easy to unpack and store, you won't waste time in setting up or taking down the equipment.

Parachute games encompass a wide range of activity levels. Parachutes work well for noisy, physical games or for quiet ones. The smallest group of people we have ever seen play together with a parachute is two. A large parachute starts to become crowded at around 40 players.

One important characteristic of parachute games is that players of different abilities, sizes, and ages can play together. This means that parachute games are perfect for families and at events such as community festivals where everyone is invited to play. Parachute games also work well in coed physical education classes. At Special Olympics events, the spectators can play right along with the Olympians.

Parachute Play Is Creative

Parachutes lend themselves to imagination. The chance to play with a 30-foot (9.1-meter) diameter swatch of colorful fabric does not come often to most people. This rare sight triggers our creative senses. As a result we are ready to become alligators, treasure hunters, cats, robbers, or other characters. In addition, this huge, billowing fabric can turn into a cloud, swamp, ocean, or igloo.

The Leader Can Play, Too

One of the great things about parachute games is that the leader also gets a chance to play. In many other types of games, the leader is more of an authority figure and must remain outside the game to act as a referee. The rules and the outcomes of these other games take on such importance that people feel better if a nonplayer watches to determine if the game is being played correctly. Because we don't keep score in most parachute games, no one has to worry about who won or whether people are playing by the rules.

Behavioral problems that might be amplified by a teacher's position of authority are defused when that interaction changes into just two players talking to each other. Some teachers have explained that this new role of fellow player allowed them an opportunity to relate to problem students in a new, more positive way. These teachers were able to carry this new style of interaction beyond the play session and make some progress in their teacher–student relationships.

Parachutes Are Cost Effective

Considering the potential number and diversity of players that can participate in and enjoy the games, parachutes are a great investment. A good, full-sized parachute costs less than $200. With proper care, a parachute that is used regularly should last for years. To complement your parachute, you might want to get some low-cost items such as foam rubber balls, Frisbees, ropes, and a large beach ball.

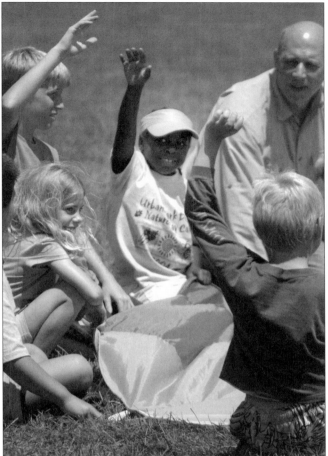

The leader of a parachute games session can do more than just explain the game—the leader gets to have fun, too!

Summary

Although there's no doubt that parachute games are fun, you can also derive a multitude of benefits from this form of play. We can actually practice cooperation, have fun, and end up with everybody feeling like a winner regardless of age, size, or ability. Through imagination we can assume many different roles and, with the parachute, can travel to exciting places. And the leader can join in the fun, too. In short, we think that a parachute is the most exciting, useful, imaginative, and versatile piece of play equipment for groups that we've ever come across.

Leading
Parachute Games

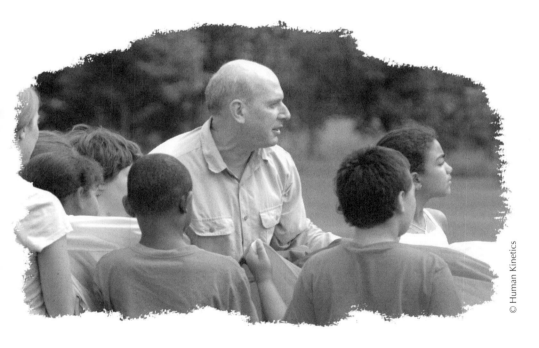

It's not enough just to throw out a parachute and a couple of sponge rubber balls and expect that people will begin playing all these parachute games on their own. Most players will discover the game of Popcorn, but nearly all the other games require some explanation and leadership. This chapter discusses how to plan and lead a parachute play session.

Leading parachute games is different from leading more traditional and well-known games such as baseball or basketball. First, the rules for parachute games are not as widely known as the rules for more traditional games. Second, the leader imparts the excitement and joy of the games to the players. This section begins with some ideas on how to be an effective, enthusiastic parachute play leader.

Leading in the Spirit of Play

As the leader, your role is to make sure that the game is not only played correctly but is also played well. A game is played correctly when all the rules are followed. A game is played well when the game is played safely and all the participants are having fun.

Making sure that the group plays a game correctly sometimes requires the leader to be a referee, especially when scores are important. (We rarely keep score when playing with a parachute.) Having an agreed-upon impartial authority frees the players to concentrate on their roles in the game without worrying about how everyone else is behaving.

Scores sometimes are kept with parachute games (such as in World Record Merry-Go-Round), but only if it enhances play. Rather than concentrating on who won, the leader's main role is to ensure that everyone has an enjoyable time. This shifts the leader's focus to whether the game is being played well, that is, to ensuring that everyone has fun and that the play environment is safe. The best way to know if a game is both fun and safe is to be a fellow player in the game. Playing along in the game gives a much different perspective than refereeing the game from the outside. If you are having fun as you play the game, it is likely that the other players are also having fun. If you are bored, it is likely that the others are bored, too.

As long as everyone is enjoying the game and having a good time, then by all means keep on playing. When interest in a game begins to wane, switch to a different game or put the parachute away for another time. Leave people with a sense of how much fun it is to play with a parachute, and they will look forward to the next opportunity to play with it. As with most games, if you play too long, people's enthusiasm is likely to fade, and they may not look forward to a future parachute play session.

Planning the Play Session

Before the play session begins, give some thought to how much time you have for the session, who will be playing, and where you will be playing. All these factors will help you choose appropriate games. As you play and become more familiar with parachute games, you will develop a sense of how long a game stays fun and which games are appropriate for which settings.

A play session with a parachute can last from 5 to 50 minutes. We don't recommend planning a 50-minute play session the first time you bring out a parachute, though. Give both your players and yourself a chance to get used to the subtlety and nuances of parachute play before you attempt such a long session.

Selecting the Playing Field

The best place to play with a parachute is outdoors on a level, grassy field. However, we don't always have these ideal conditions or even a choice of venue. Fortunately, you can play with a parachute indoors as well as outdoors. Just make sure you have enough room. Also, don't forget the height of the ceiling when choosing your play space. Balls launched from a parachute can soar pretty high.

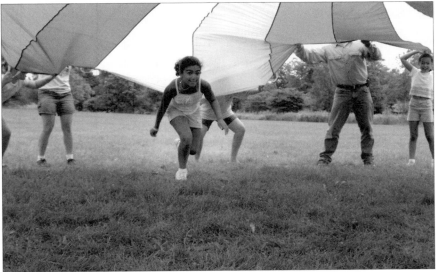

© Human Kinetics

While not necessary, a grassy field is an ideal playing surface for parachute games.

Your playing field will help you decide which games to play. For example, it is best to play Parachute Ride and Alligator on a nice, freshly waxed, slippery, wooden gym floor. While not necessary, a slippery floor makes it easier for Alligators to pull victims into the swamp. This same slippery condition might make it dangerous to play a running game such as Heartbeat. When special considerations need to be made, we make recommendations on the best type of playing field for the games in the descriptions.

Make a List of Games

The best piece of advice we give all play leaders is to write down a list of games and keep it handy whenever you lead a play session. This gives you something to fall back on if you draw a blank while trying to think of the next game. As you read through this book and become familiar with the games, make a list of the ones you think will work the best for your situation.

Having a list is so important to us that we had T-shirts printed with a giant games list for the New Games workshops we conducted for community play-festival leaders. But we made a mistake by printing the list right side up, which meant the text appeared upside down to the wearer. More than once during a festival, excited play leaders asked strangers to read their shirts to them.

It is very reassuring to have your list of games handy. When you get swept up in the spirit of play and forget everything you planned, you will be able to reach in your pocket, pull out your list, and choose the next game. We usually lead play sessions that include both parachute and nonparachute games, so our games lists include more than just the games in this book. We categorize the games in several ways that are important to us. We categorize the games according to activity level (low, medium, or high), number of players, or timing (good beginning, middle, or end games). These categories will help you identify the most appropriate games for almost any situation.

Making sure your list includes only the good games that you and your fellow players know and enjoy helps you lead fun play sessions. In other words, this should be a personal list just for you. Please don't just copy down a list of games from a book, not even from this book. You may want to write down a list of games in the order that you want to play them for a specific session. This will certainly add to your confidence as the play leader. Don't be afraid, however, to veer from this predetermined order of games if a better idea appears during the actual play session. Remember that a large component of play is being spontaneous.

During the Play Session

Executing a play session with a parachute is easy. You need to plan only three things: how to begin, how to end, and what to do in the middle.

Getting Started

Starting a play session with a parachute is easy. Roll out the parachute and have everyone grab an edge. Make sure that the players roll the edge in a few times and tuck their fingers under the roll for a good grip. This will also protect the perimeter of the parachute. Some parachutes come with handles, which means the players don't even have to roll up the edge. They just grab on to the handles. Other parachutes have a special rope sewn into the edge to make it easier for players to grab the parachute.

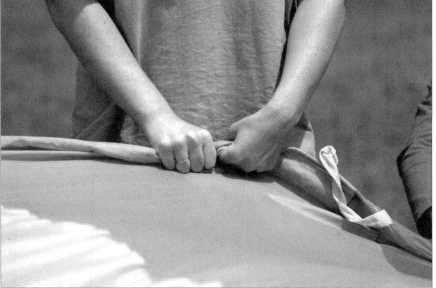

© Human Kinetics

If your parachute doesn't have a rope sewn into the edge for a nice handhold, have the players roll the edge in a few times to give themselves a better grip.

Locating and Fetching Equipment and Introducing Ideas

One important job of a play leader is to provide the needed equipment at the right time, so sometimes your role is that of gofer. The game of Popcorn requires foam balls, and you are the one to retrieve them. Have extra sponge balls, Frisbees, and ropes in a duffel bag nearby but out of the way until you need them. It's also very easy to delegate this job to other players if you like. We have found that designating reluctant or disruptive players as gofers usually helps bring them into the game.

A play leader is often a gofer for the rules, too. Because you are the one who knows how to play the game, you are the leader.

Selecting Teams

Need to split up into two teams? How about players born in the first six months of the year versus players born in the last six months of the year? Or you can pit everyone born on an even day of the month against all those born on odd days. You can group astrological signs together into teams or against one another. Or you can say, "All players wearing the color blue over there and everyone else over here." We sometimes ask players to instantly raise one hand high with either one or two fingers extended. Keeping their hands up, they must find all their teammates who are showing the same number of fingers. Sometimes one or two players change their fingers because they want to be on the same team as a friend. That's okay with us.

In many parachute games the players are already standing around the edge of the chute. You can quickly make two teams by designating any diameter of the chute as the equator. Dividing the parachute into a northern and southern hemisphere instantly creates two teams.

Choosing Volunteers for Special Roles

Kids have a hard time when it comes to picking volunteers. They don't have a well-developed sense of how to wait. If they are not chosen right away, they become frustrated. Instead of asking for volunteers, we try to be more creative.

For instance, we hold spontaneous lotteries to pick our volunteers. We might announce that anyone who is wearing polka dots should go into the middle for Sculpture. After the first round, the art pieces get to pick their replacements, but they must pick players who have not already had a turn. Be careful about calling out, "Blue jeans," to choose someone. That's a great way to pick over half of your group as volunteers. By the way, kids notice if you aren't being fair, so be careful about playing favorites.

Just as it is possible to divide into teams by birthdays, you can choose volunteers this way: "Anyone born in the month of May goes into the middle for the next round." You can group months together if you like, or you can even choose people by seasons if it is appropriate. Sometimes kids will claim they have multiple birthdays so that they can get into the middle several times, but this usually isn't a major problem.

You can also stand in the middle, close your eyes, and spin around with your arm extended. When you stop, simply open your eyes, see where your arm is pointing, and choose the nearest person with a raised arm.

Unlike kids, adults are usually reluctant to volunteer. As we get older, most of us are increasingly unwilling to take risks or look foolish, especially in front of others. If you, as play leader, are willing to be a volunteer, it shows others that there is no reason to be afraid, and the adult players will be more willing to volunteer for the next game.

Keeping Things Fun

Along with all the other responsibilities, a frequent role of the leader is that of enthusiasm creator, someone who knows the rules and gets the game going in such a way that people want to join in, expecting a fun

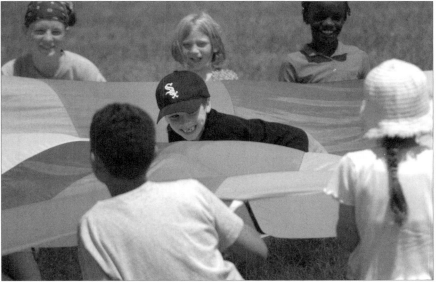

© Human Kinetics

The best rule to remember when leading a parachute game is to have fun!

time. Enthusiasm is contagious. If you enjoy what you are doing and you let it show, other people will want to try it also.

Hold a Practice Round

Having a hard time persuading people to try out a new game? To get people to start playing before they fully understand the rules, we allow them to play a practice round. Because practice doesn't really count, people are willing to try the game, even though they may not really understand it. A practice round frequently stops players from asking irrelevant questions before the game begins. During a practice round of Interlocking Gears, people can see for themselves where the gears mesh. You won't have to explain it several times.

There is something about not wanting to lose that makes most people wary about trying something they don't fully understand. But you can't lose a practice round; it's only practice. Actually, it is hard to lose at any parachute game. We don't have losers; we have players. We typically don't keep score, and we don't give out trophies at the end of the session. Take away the external rewards of scores and prizes, and it doesn't matter if people are just practicing or are really playing. Sometimes at the beginning, it helps people to think of playing as only practicing.

The important thing is to have fun. We have found that people have more fun actually doing things than listening to instructions on how to do things. We try to get the games going as quickly as possible, even if it means there is sometimes a little bit of confusion at the start. Calling it "practice" lets people feel okay about going through the motions before understanding everything. If it is a good game, people will figure it out soon enough.

Varying the Game

Feel free to modify these games to better suit your group and your environment. We provide some examples of how to change games in the Variations category of each game. Our hope is that these ideas will lead you to create even more adaptations and variations.

As a general rule, any game that involves walking or running can also have the players jump, jog, skip, walk backward, hop on one leg, crawl, or perform any other appropriate means of locomotion.

Discipline When Necessary

If some of your players are acting up, then it is your job to make sure they do not disrupt the game. In this case your role may be one of an authority figure. Part of your job as the teacher or activity leader is to keep the focus. There may be no one perfect way of responding to disruptive behavior. Kids often feel a need to test you to see what you will do in a given situation. We have found that responding fairly and even-handedly is best.

One approach we use is to tell disruptive players to sit out for a game. We tell them that they are welcome to return to the next game if they can keep from disrupting it. We have found it is important not to explain this in anger. With anger, we only get more resistance. If you do need to tell more than one person to sit out, it's best to have them sit separately. Playing with a parachute is so much fun that people want to play rather than sit out. Putting the responsibility for participation on the players is a tactic that usually works.

Ensuring Safety

Since safety is such an overriding concern, this section covers a range of safety issues.

Physical Safety

Most parachute games are inherently safe. Everyone standing in a circle looking at one another creates an awareness of the group that reinforces

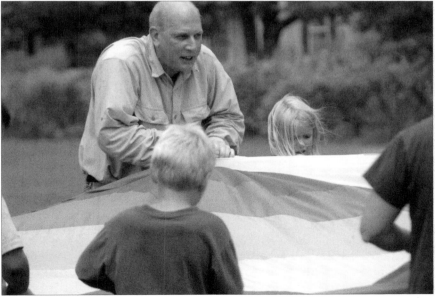

As the leader of parachute games, you have the responsibility to keep the game safe and make sure the participants are playing appropriately.

people's concerns for each other's safety. Also, few games involve aggressive contact. However, as leader you always have the responsibility to see that no one gets hurt. It's up to you to keep the game from getting out of control. Being a participant in the game gives you a sense of when the game is starting to become too wild and unsafe.

If you think that the game is unsafe, stop it or change to a milder version of the same game. A milder version of Cat and Mouse, for example, places the cats down on all fours instead of running around on top of the parachute. One of the great things about parachute games is that everyone wants to play them over and over again. This is not true if someone gets injured. An injured player will have to recuperate before she or he can play again, and the entire group tends to get dispirited after an accident.

Again, parachute games are safe. We dislike injuries so much that we are taking time here to help you avoid silly accidents. In the descriptions of the games, we point out the few minor safety problems. For example, when playing Racing Heartbeat, some people may want to bring the parachute down too quickly on their fellow players. Just point out that there is a steady rhythm to the game, and the object is not to decapitate each other. We also remind people who are changing positions to avoid collisions by watching out for others as they run across.

Notice that we don't even suggest using a parachute to toss people up into the air. When done safely, this can certainly be a fun activity. However, we can't personally inspect everyone's parachute for strength. Keep in mind that parachutes wear out. A parachute that was great for tossing people last summer may have become too fragile for that purpose this year. Such an activity also puts a great strain on the stitching, causing the parachute to come apart at the seams or even tear.

We discussed whether or not we should have a special section explaining how to toss folks safely. Then we thought about liability insurance. Then we thought about someone being confined to a wheelchair as a result of one quick, cheap thrill on a parachute. Rather than risk a potential injury by having someone accidentally fall through a parachute, we would just as soon not use, and encourage you not to use, a parachute for tossing people.

Emotional Safety

A leader needs to be sensitive to the players' emotional safety when playing with a parachute as well as when playing other games. Many people have never played with a parachute before and will feel uncertain about their roles in the games. Your job as play leader is to invite them into the game and help them feel welcome. You can involve bystanders by just pointing out a gap somewhere on the edge of the parachute and saying, "We could use a few more people over here." On the one hand, don't insist that people play; they should always have the option to sit out. On the other hand, do invite them in and make them feel comfortable about joining. Many people need to be sure they are welcome, so you might have to extend several invitations. Playful coaxing is a fun, rewarding activity in itself.

Once people are in the game, make sure that they don't feel they are being singled out or picked on. We try not to ask for just one volunteer at a time. That way no one feels completely isolated and put in the spotlight. You might want to keep this in mind, though parachute games rarely use solo volunteers. The only game in this book that involves asking someone to do something alone is Cat and Mouse. But even then, at least two players, the cat and the mouse, participate at the same time. We have found that the spirit of play is enhanced when people get to do things together. Most folks get nervous when we ask them to step outside the group and do something risky, such as try to guess what everybody else is thinking. They feel better if they have at least one partner to help them guess.

Our feelings about safety can be summarized as follows: Parachute games are so much fun we want people to be able to play them over and over again. If they suffer a physical injury, they won't be able to play anymore. If they get too embarrassed, they won't want to play anymore. The group will also be less inclined to participate if they see these things happening to their fellow players.

Summary

The leader knows the rules and creates the mood. The responsibility for making sure that things go smoothly and that transitions from one game to the next are timely and appropriate for the feeling of the group rests on the leader. Other responsibilities include letting everyone feel welcome and safe. Best of all, after explaining the game, the leader becomes a player and leads only when necessary. This last quality is how the parachute play leader differs from a play leader in more traditional sports and recreational games. In the next chapter, we will look at the skills that are an inherent part of the games.

Enhancing Developmental Skills

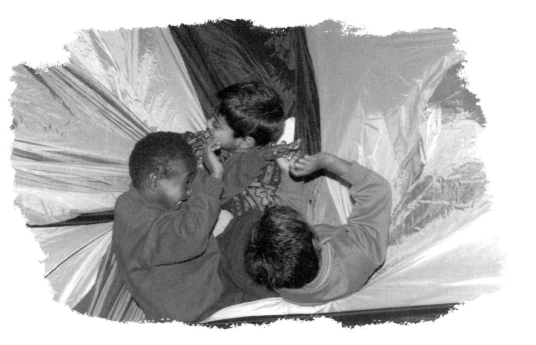

A child's development involves acquiring certain social, personal, motor, and perceptual skills during his or her daily activities. As children get older, they generally grow bigger, stronger, more agile, and more coordinated. Not everyone acquires these skills at the same rate or to the same degree. Sometimes it becomes painfully obvious that a child has not mastered a skill that is simple for most.

Individual differences account for a number of variances in the rate of development. There are three primary factors:

1. Children develop coordination at different rates.
2. Neurological problems account for some variances.
3. Lack of opportunity to practice skills explains other differences.

Parachute games can be useful for this third situation, providing an occasion to improve skills in a way that is fun and exciting.

The games presented in this book aren't intended primarily for developing skills. The focus is on playing and having fun. People don't play to develop skills. However, the games do help players improve their

- social skills,
- personal behavior,
- perceptual and physical skills, and
- basic motor skills.

Social Skills

Parachute games expose people to several social skills, including skills related to cooperation, trust, problem solving, communication, physical touching, and adaptability. Through the years we have seen people grow in and develop their social skills through participation in games. In this section we look at specific social skills and suggest games that use and develop these skills. You can then go to the games finder on pages vii to viii to locate the page numbers of each game.

Cooperation

The following games feature the skill of working together for a common goal:

- Alligator
- Ball Surfing
- Big Bang
- Blow Up
- Cat and Mouse
- Circular Sit-Ups
- Climb the Mountain
- Cop and Robber
- Floating Mushroom
- Flying Parachute

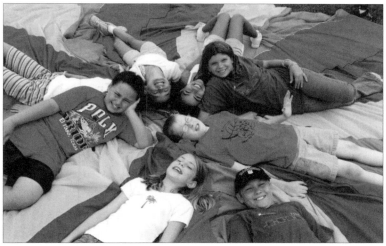

Photo courtesy of Ragen E. Sanner

Parachute games are a lot of fun and they help to develop an array of social skills.

- Free Play
- Ghost Rider
- Group Balance
- Heartbeat
- Housekeeping
- Igloo
- Interlocking Gears
- Jumbo Mushroom
- Liftoff
- Missile Launch
- Mushroom
- Ostrich
- Parachute Basketball
- Parachute Golf
- Parachute Volleyball
- Popovers
- Rabbit and Hound
- Racing Heartbeat
- Rocking Chair
- Sculpture
- Shark
- Swooping Cloud
- Turnover
- Wave Wall
- Who's Peeking?

These games include cooperation as a part of their activity:

- Centipede
- Circular Tug
- Dodge 'Em
- I Dare Ya
- It's in the Bag
- Jell-O
- Jellyfish Jaunt
- Wave Machine
- Merry-Go-Round
- Over Under
- Pony Express
- Treasure Hunt
- Waves Overhead
- World Record Merry-Go-Round

Trust

The following games involve building a feeling of group safety:

- Circular Tug
- Cop and Robber
- Group Balance
- Liftoff
- Racing Heartbeat
- Sculpture
- Wave Rolling

Problem Solving

The following games feature problem solving as a major characteristic:

- Free Play
- Over Under
- Sculpture

These games have problem solving as one feature:

- Cop and Robber
- Cover Up
- Dodge 'Em
- Housekeeping
- I Dare Ya
- Parachute Volleyball
- Rabbit and Hound
- Treasure Hunt
- Turnover
- Wave Rolling

Verbal Contact

The following games use interaction with speech (including listening skills) as a major characteristic:

- Ghost Rider
- Group Balance
- Over Under
- Turnover

These games involve some speaking and listening:

- Alligator
- Ball Surfing
- Cat and Mouse
- Circular Tug
- Climb the Mountain
- Cop and Robber
- Dodge 'Em
- Floating Mushroom

- Flying Parachute
- Housekeeping
- I Dare Ya
- Igloo
- Interlocking Gears
- Jell-O
- Jellyfish Jaunt
- Jumbo Mushroom
- Liftoff
- Merry-Go-Round
- Mushroom
- Parachute Golf
- Parachute Volleyball
- Pony Express
- Popovers
- Rabbit and Hound
- Raceway
- Racing Heartbeat
- Sculpture
- Shark
- Swooping Cloud
- Treasure Hunt
- Wave Wall
- Who's Peeking?
- World Record Merry-Go-Round

Tactile Contact

All of the games include physical contact with the parachute. These particular games require touching other people:

- Alligator
- Cat and Mouse
- Free Play
- Pony Express
- Sculpture
- Shark
- Turnover

Touching other people is one feature of the following games:

- Climb the Mountain
- Cop and Robber
- Gophers
- I Dare Ya
- Jell-O
- Parachute Pass
- Racing Heartbeat
- Top of the Pops
- Wave Rolling
- Waves Overhead

Adaptability

In this context, *adaptability* refers to how a person's responses fit the actions and movements of others. Following are games that require a high degree of adaptability.

- Cop and Robber
- Dodge 'Em
- Gophers
- Heartbeat
- Housekeeping
- Igloo
- Jumbo Mushroom
- Mushroom
- Racing Heartbeat
- Rocking Chair
- Turnover
- Wave Rolling

Adaptability is also one property of the following games:

- Alligator
- Ball Surfing
- Centipede
- Circular Sit-Ups
- Circular Tug
- Floating Mushroom
- Flying Parachute
- Free Play
- Ghost Rider
- Group Balance
- I Dare Ya
- Jellyfish Jaunt
- Merry-Go-Round
- Over Under
- Parachute Golf
- Parachute Pass
- Parachute Volleyball
- Popovers
- Rabbit and Hound
- Raceway
- Sculpture
- Shark
- Snake Tag
- Treasure Hunt
- Wave Wall
- World Record Merry-Go-Round

Personal Behavior

The skills of personal behavior considered here are self-control, creativity, spontaneity, and pantomime.

Self-Control

The following games involve aspects of self-control:

- Gophers
- Housekeeping
- I Dare Ya
- Missile Launch
- Parachute Basketball
- Sculpture
- Top of the Pops
- Treasure Hunt

Self-control plays a smaller role in these games:

- Alligator
- Ball Surfing
- Big Bang
- Cat and Mouse
- Circular Sit-Ups
- Circular Tug
- Cop and Robber
- Cover Up
- Dodge 'Em
- Drag Race
- Floating Mushroom
- Flying Parachute
- Ghost Rider
- Group Balance
- Igloo
- Interlocking Gears
- It's in the Bag
- Jellyfish Jaunt
- Jumbo Mushroom
- Liftoff
- Merry-Go-Round
- Mushroom
- Ostrich
- Parachute Pass
- Parachute Volleyball
- Pony Express
- Popcorn
- Popovers
- Rabbit and Hound
- Raceway
- Racing Heartbeat
- Rocking Chair
- Shark
- Snake Tag
- Wave Machine
- Wave Rolling
- Waves Overhead
- Who's Peeking?
- World Record Merry-Go-Round

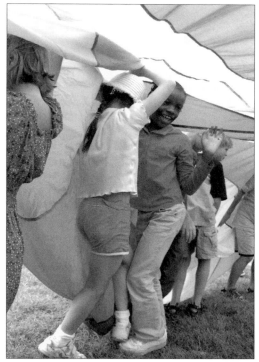

© Human Kinetics

Parachute games allow for a fun way to explore personal behavior and self-control.

Creativity

These games require the players to use ideas inventively:

- Free Play
- Sculpture

Creativity is a minor feature of the following games:

- Cover Up
- I Dare Ya
- It's in the Bag
- Racing Heartbeat
- Turnover
- Wave Rolling

Spontaneity

A notable element of these games is impromptu action in the absence of specific instructions:

- Alligator
- Dodge 'Em
- Free Play
- Sculpture
- Shark
- Turnover
- Who's Peeking?

Spontaneity is also a factor in the following games:

- Blow Up
- Cat and Mouse
- Centipede
- Circular Tug
- Cover Up
- Gophers
- Housekeeping
- I Dare Ya
- Jellyfish Jaunt
- Parachute Pass
- Parachute Ride
- Popcorn
- Popovers
- Top of the Pops
- Wave Rolling

Pantomime

In the following games, an important part is expression through acting movements:

- Alligator
- Shark

Some acting movements are required in the following games:

- Cop and Robber
- Dodge 'Em
- It's in the Bag
- Jell-O

Perceptual and Physical Skills

The elements in perceptual and physical skills are visual ability, skillfulness, coordination, reaction, strength, and endurance.

Visual Ability

These games call for observation and peripheral perception:

- Ball Surfing
- Cat and Mouse
- Cop and Robber
- Dodge 'Em
- Gophers
- Housekeeping
- Jell-O
- Missile Launch
- Over Under
- Parachute Basketball
- Rabbit and Hound
- Racing Heartbeat
- Top of the Pops
- Treasure Hunt
- Who's Peeking?

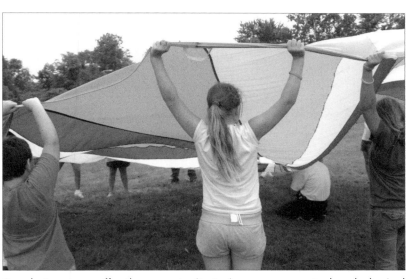

Parachute games offer the opportunity to improve perceptual and physical skills.

Although not an absolute necessity, visual ability is helpful for the following games:

- Centipede
- Circular Tug
- Climb the Mountain
- Floating Mushroom
- Flying Parachute
- Free Play
- Ghost Rider
- Group Balance
- Heartbeat
- I Dare Ya
- Igloo
- Interlocking Gears
- It's in the Bag
- Jellyfish Jaunt
- Jumbo Mushroom
- Liftoff
- Mushroom
- Parachute Golf
- Parachute Pass
- Parachute Ride
- Parachute Volleyball
- Pony Express
- Popcorn
- Popovers
- Raceway
- Sculpture
- Shark
- Snake Tag
- Swooping Cloud
- Wave Rolling
- Wave Wall

Skillfulness and Coordination

These games require complex body movements:

- Ghost Rider
- Gophers
- Igloo
- It's in the Bag
- Pony Express
- Treasure Hunt

These games also involve complex body movements, but to a lesser degree:

- Dodge 'Em
- Drag Race
- I Dare Ya
- It's in the Bag
- Jell-O
- Merry-Go-Round
- Missile Launch
- Ostrich
- Parachute Basketball
- Parachute Pass
- Rocking Chair
- Top of the Pops
- Who's Peeking?
- World Record Merry-Go-Round

Reaction

The games here call for a quick physical response:

- Ball Surfing
- Cat and Mouse
- Climb the Mountain
- Cop and Robber
- Drag Race
- Floating Mushroom
- Flying Parachute
- Gophers
- I Dare Ya
- Parachute Pass
- Popovers
- Top of the Pops
- Treasure Hunt
- Who's Peeking?

These games also need quick reactions, but to a lesser extent:

- Big Bang
- Ghost Rider
- Missile Launch
- Over Under
- Parachute Basketball
- Pony Express
- Popcorn
- Rabbit and Hound
- Snake Tag
- Swooping Cloud
- Wave Wall
- World Record Merry-Go-Round

Strength

These games require strength in the upper body. They all involve lifting:

- Heartbeat
- Housekeeping
- Liftoff
- Parachute Ride
- Rabbit and Hound
- Racing Heartbeat
- Snake Tag
- Top of the Pops
- Wave Machine
- Wave Rolling
- Waves Overhead

Strength is one of the elements of the following games:

- Alligator
- Ball Surfing
- Big Bang
- Cat and Mouse
- Circular Sit-Ups
- Circular Tug
- Floating Mushroom
- Flying Parachute

- Ghost Rider
- Jumbo Mushroom
- Mushroom
- Parachute Golf
- Parachute Volleyball

- Popcorn
- Popovers
- Swooping Cloud
- Wave Wall

Endurance

The ability to continue the activity is important here:

- Flying Parachute
- I Dare Ya
- Jellyfish Jaunt
- Popcorn

- Raceway
- Wave Machine
- Wave Rolling
- Waves Overhead

These games require some endurance:

- Cat and Mouse
- Housekeeping
- Merry-Go-Round
- Popovers
- Rabbit and Hound

- Snake Tag
- Top of the Pops
- World Record Merry-Go-Round

Basic Motor Skills

The basic motor skills involved in these games are walking, running, jumping, balancing, leaning, crawling, hopping, and throwing and catching.

Walking

Walking is a major part in these games:

- Interlocking Gears
- Merry-Go-Round

Walking is also a part of these games:

- Centipede
- Jumbo Mushroom
- Over Under

- Parachute Ride
- Shark

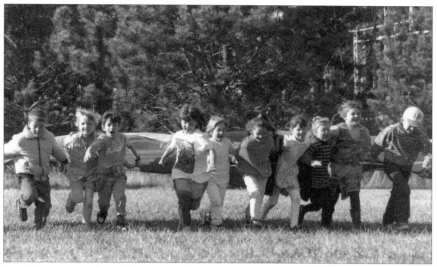

Parachutes games are a fun way to develop basic motor skills.

Running

Running is important in the following games:

- Cop and Robber
- Flying Parachute
- Jellyfish Jaunt
- Raceway
- World Record Merry-Go-Round

Running is a part of the following games:

- Housekeeping
- I Dare Ya
- It's in the Bag
- Parachute Basketball
- Racing Heartbeat
- Treasure Hunt

Jumping

Jumping is an integral skill for these games:

- Merry-Go-Round
- World Record Merry-Go-Round

Jumping is an element of these games:

- Dodge 'Em
- It's in the Bag
- Jell-O
- Parachute Basketball

Balancing

An ability to maintain balance is crucial for this game:

- Group Balance

Maintaining balance is a skill used in these games as well:

- Circular Tug
- Free Play
- Merry-Go-Round
- Parachute Ride
- Pony Express
- Sculpture
- Turnover
- World Record Merry-Go-Round

Leaning

These games call for leaning:

- Cat and Mouse
- Circular Tug
- Group Balance
- Pony Express

To a lesser extent, leaning is also used in these games:

- Alligator
- Cop and Robber
- Sculpture

Crawling

These games involve crawling on the hands and knees or on the belly:

- Alligator
- Cat and Mouse
- Climb the Mountain
- Free Play
- Gophers
- Jell-O
- Pony Express
- Top of the Pops
- Wave Rolling

Hopping

These games may feature hopping on one foot:

- Merry-Go-Round
- World Record Merry-Go-Round

These games can also include hopping:

- I Dare Ya
- Jell-O

Throwing and Catching

These are games in which throwing and catching are part of the activity:

- Dodge 'Em
- Gophers
- Housekeeping
- Missile Launch
- Parachute Basketball
- Top of the Pops

Throwing and catching can be involved in this game, too:

- Popcorn

Choosing and Caring for Your Parachute

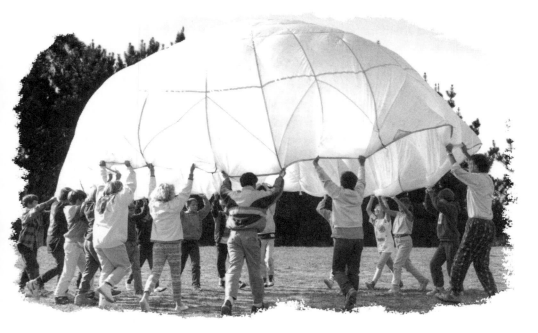

So far, so good. You know the benefits of parachute play, and you know how to lead the games and how games help develop specific skills. If you don't yet have a parachute, don't know where to find one, or don't know what to look for when purchasing one, you've come to the right chapter. We will cover these topics and more.

Purchasing Your Parachute

When people purchase diamonds, they are frequently advised to learn about the four Cs: color, clarity, cut, and caret. Some folks add a fifth C, cost.

After spending a few minutes with a thesaurus, we found that a similar set of guideline Cs can be used for purchasing a parachute: circumference, color, construction, and constitution. Again, the fifth C would be cost.

Circumference

This has to do with the size of the parachute. The circumference is the perimeter, or outside edge, of a circle. All points on the circumference of a circle are equidistant from the center.

Rather than listing the circumference, most parachute manufacturers size their chutes in terms of the diameter. A diameter is a straight line that connects two opposite points of the circumference and passes through the center. The relationship between the circumference and the diameter is expressed in the equation $D \times \pi = C$. Multiply the diameter by pi (3.14), and you can determine the circumference.

Perhaps more important than knowing the circumference of your parachute is knowing how big of a chute you need for the number of players you have. If you use a parachute that has handles, and the handles are an integral part of the games, then the question is answered quite easily: Choose a parachute that has enough handles for each player. (Note: Handles are discussed later in the Constitution section.)

Those who use parachutes without handles should estimate that each foot (about 30.5 centimeters) of diameter translates into about one player along the circumference. A 20-foot (6.1-meter) diameter parachute will be good for about 20 players. A 24-foot (7.3-meter) diameter chute is good for about 24 players. Of course, these are just general guidelines. You can fit more small players around the edge of a parachute than you can large players. You can also have more people around the edge if they are friendly and don't mind squishing in a bit.

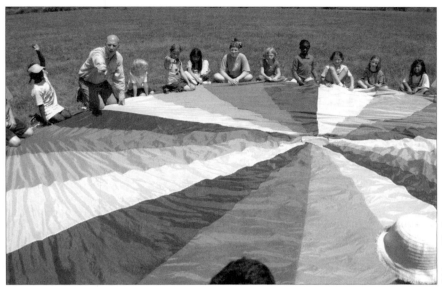

© Human Kinetics

The bright colors and patterns available on today's parachutes help create an exciting environment, as well as provide visual cues for some of the games.

Color

How would you like your parachute decorated? Long gone are the days of buying an all-white, army-surplus parachute. Today's play chutes offer a large number of choices. Play chutes with brightly colored panels are the norm. Additionally, manufacturers are designing play chutes with smiling faces, letters and numbers, and other designs.

The advantage of being able to refer to the colored panels to create teams and designate individual players in games such as Rabbit and Hound, Racing Heartbeat, Popcorn, and others sways us into preferring parachutes with colored panels. If you have particular reasons to choose a parachute with a specific design, then by all means be comfortable with that choice.

Construction

How well is the parachute made? The two factors to be aware of are quality of the material and how the material is sewn together.

Most parachutes are made of ripstop nylon. Some are made of polyester. In both cases the weight of the material is measured by its denier number. A higher denier number for a parachute means the chute will be heavier, stronger, and usually more expensive than a same-size parachute with a lower denier number. For example, a parachute using fabric with a denier rating of 70 is lighter than a parachute with a denier rating of 250.

For many parachutes the fabric is chain-stitched together. Although chain stitching is fine, lock stitching is even better. If thread that has been chain-stitched breaks, then it is more likely that the remaining thread will unravel than if the thread had been lock-stitched. Lock stitching locks in each stitch, which helps prevent broken threads from unraveling.

A one-year warranty against rips and tears acquired during normal use is standard. Some warranties are longer. Longer warranties are usually indications that the parachute is made of a higher-denier material and has better stitching.

With shipping and handling charges added to the labor and materials required to repair a parachute, it is often easier to replace an out-of-warranty parachute rather than to have one returned, repaired, and shipped back.

Constitution

This term covers the various parts of a parachute, such as center hole, mesh, handles, circumference rope, and portholes. Is there a hole in the center, or is there mesh? Our preference is to have an open hole, as several of the games involve balls passing through the center hole.

In the first edition of *Parachute Games,* we wrote, "It is our experience that even when the handles are sewn on securely, they tend to be the first section of the parachute to deteriorate." We are happy to say that many of the parachute manufacturers have become aware of and fixed this problem. Many parachutes today have a strong rope sewn into the perimeter of the parachute. The handles are sewn to this rope, not just to the fabric of the parachute. If you would like a chute with handles that last, make sure that the handles are sewn to the rope and not just to the fabric.

Also on the topic of handles, we have occasionally seen parachutes with handles that were made by having a bounding perimeter rope that was shorter in length than the circumference of the parachute. These were not good play parachutes. The shorter length, or smaller circumference, of the bounding rope meant that the players could never pull the parachute taut to be entirely flat. Excess fabric limited many of the games that could be played, such as Popcorn, Snake Tag, Liftoff, and others. We finally got rid of the handles by cutting the bounding rope. The result was a vast improvement. The parachute was only slightly less strong. The chute was also free to be pulled taut and was more fun to play with. Our advice is to avoid parachutes that have a bounding perimeter rope whose circumference is less than the circumference of the spread-out parachute.

One exciting new development in the constitution of parachutes, as mentioned previously, is the folding and sewing of the edge of the parachute over a strong rope around the circumference, with the rope sewn in place. This makes for a stronger parachute and also provides a better grip for players to hold on to the edge. This feature will probably add some cost to your chute. Although it is not necessary, we think you should consider this type of parachute if your budget can handle it.

Another new development is the creation of portholes in parachutes. Portholes are holes cut in the fabric and covered with mesh. Portholes let you see what's going on inside of the parachute, in addition to letting players underneath the chute see what is going on outside. Portholes also make for a brighter environment underneath the parachute, since the mesh lets in more light than regular fabric. If you work with extremely young or boisterous children, you may want to consider a parachute with portholes. The extra security of being able to keep your eyes on both the interior and exterior of the parachute can be well worth the cost.

Distributors

Type the words *play* and *parachute* into any decent Internet search engine, and you will find many more suppliers of parachutes than can be listed here. Following are some reputable parachute supply companies with which we have had experience. Many of these suppliers use the same manufacturer, so the parachutes are the same.

Companies are listed alphabetically with their current addresses, phone numbers, and Web sites as of this writing. Of course, all this information is subject to change. Please contact the suppliers for their most recent prices and product updates.

North America

Childcraft Education Corporation
P.O. Box 3239
Lancaster, PA 17604
800-631-5652
www.childcrafteducation.com

FlagHouse
601 FlagHouse Dr.
Hasbrouck Heights, NJ 07604-3116
800-793-7900
www.flaghouse.com

Front Row Experience
540 Discovery Bay Blvd.
Discovery Bay, CA 94514
800-524-9091
www.frontrowexperience.com

Gopher Sport
220 24th Ave. Northwest
P.O. Box 998
Owatonna, MN 55060
800-533-0446
www.gophersport.com

According to a company representative, Gopher Sport offers a lifetime warranty on all of its equipment, including parachutes.

Great Lakes Sports
P.O. Box 447
Lambertville, MI 48144
800-446-2114
www.greatlakessports.com

Lakeshore Learning Materials
2695 E. Dominguez St.
Carson, CA 90895
800-778-4456
www.lakeshorelearning.com

Morley Athletic Supply Company, Inc.
P.O. Box 557
208 Division St.
Amsterdam, NY 12010
800-811-1931
www.morleyathletic.com

NASCO
901 Janesville Ave.
P.O. Box 901
Fort Atkinson, WI 53538-0901
800-558-9595
www.enasco.com

Palos Sports, Inc.
11711 S. Austin Ave.
Alsip, IL 60803
800-233-5484
www.palossports.com

Palos Sports, Inc. offers a two-year warranty on its premium line of parachutes.

Parachute Shop
Pepperell Airport
165 Nashua Rd.
Pepperell, MA 01463
800-872-2488
www.parachuteshop.com

Parachute Shop sells actual parachutes for skydiving as well as play parachutes. They also sell 2-inch by 25-foot (5.08-centimeter by 7.62-meter) rolls of ripstop parachute repair tape in many different colors. Additionally, they are the only company we currently know of that repairs parachutes.

S&S Worldwide
P.O. Box 513
75 Mill St.
Colchester, CT 06415
800-243-9232
www.ssww.com

School Specialty Canada
Unit 200, 5510-268 St.
Langley, BC V4W 3X4
866-519-2816
www.schoolspecialty.ca/sportime

Sportime, Inc.
3155 Northwoods Pkwy.
Norcross, GA 30071
800-444-5700
www.sportime.com

Tinker Tots
5770 E. River Valley Trail
Anaheim Hills, CA 92807
714-921-2332
www.tinkertots.com

Toledo P.E. Supply
5101 Advantage Dr.
Toledo, OH 43612
800-225-7749
www.tpesonline.com

US Games
P.O. Box 7726
Dallas, Texas 75209
800-327-0484
www.us-games.com

Wolverine Sports
745 State Circle
Box 1941
Ann Arbor, MI 48106
800-521-2832
www.wolverinesports.com

Europe

SeamStress Ltd.
23 Banbury Rd.
Byfield, Northants
NN11 6XJ, UK
Tel/Fax: [+44] (0)1327-263933
www.playchutes.com

SeamStress Ltd. custom-makes its parachutes to order.

Repairing Your Parachute

Most companies honor their warranties by replacing rather than repairing parachutes. That's great. But what do you do when you tear your out-of-warranty, more-than-one-year-old parachute? Sewing a torn parachute isn't a bad idea, although sewing one by hand is time-consuming.

An alternative to sewing is mending rips with parachute repair tape. Parachute repair tape is a light, ripstop nylon with a strong adhesive backing on one side. The tape is available in many different colors and is usually sold in 2-inch-wide (5.08-centimeter-wide) rolls. Lay your torn parachute out, match the two sides of the rip, and tape them back together.

Cleaning Your Parachute

As for washing or cleaning your parachute, the manufacturers' instructions vary considerably. One says to use a washing machine; a second agrees but recommends using a delicate cycle with cold water. Yet another says to dry-clean the parachute.

Our experience is that it is possible and sometimes necessary to clean parachutes, especially if you play with them outdoors. Use cold water and make sure the washer is large enough for the size of the parachute. A large parachute requires an industrial-size, front-loading washing machine. Hot water may shrink the stitching thread and cause the nylon to wrinkle (and generally look strange). Do not put the parachute in the dryer for the same reason. A hot dryer can actually melt the nylon. Parachutes dry quickly if hung outdoors or spread out on the grass on a mild day.

Decorating Your Parachute

If you intend to play games with your parachute, then you probably do not want to decorate it. Paint adds weight and peels off during play. However, you might like to spray-paint or silkscreen words onto your parachute

You have more decorating options if you plan to use your parachute primarily as a decoration. Fabric and acrylic paints work well with parachutes. You can purchase these paints at craft or art supply stores. Acrylic inks tend to bleed, which may create a great effect.

Storing and Caring for Your Parachute

Store your parachute in a storage bag in a dry, warm spot. Cool, moist conditions may cause mold. Keeping the parachute in its storage bag helps keep moisture out and prevents bits of the parachute from sneaking into trouble, like into that spot of grease or oil on the garage floor.

Get into the habit of stuffing your parachute into its bag. Folding the parachute precisely in the same manner each time, as for a flag, may put unnecessary stress on some of the seams.

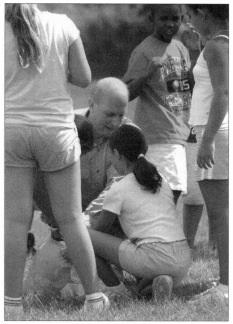

© Human Kinetics

Loosely stuff your parachute into its storage bag to keep it strong and fresh for the next play session.

Do not roll up your parachute and use it as a tug-of-war rope. We know you're thinking, *But what about Circular Tug?* This game puts an even stress on the parachute and therefore is not as harmful as the extreme stress on certain sections of a rolled-up parachute.

Summary

Now you're almost ready! You know how to get a parachute; what to look for; and how to repair, clean, decorate, and store it. But you still don't know what to do with it. Not to worry. We devote the rest of the book to games you can play with your parachute.

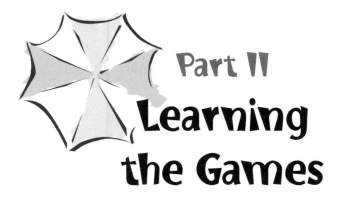

Part II
Learning the Games

Chapters 5 through 7 are the heart of this book. In them we present 59 great parachute games. Chapter 5 includes the low-activity games, chapter 6 the moderate-activity games, and chapter 7 the high-activity games. Some of the games appear in only one chapter and are classified in two categories, such as low to moderate or moderate to high. That's because these borderline games can move from one level of intensity to another, depending on how much energy you and your fellow players want to exert.

We present all the games in a format that enables you to understand quickly the requirements and possibilities of each game as you select what to play. After the game description, the following categories may appear:

Safety Tips These tips appear as a heading when there are important factors you need to be aware of in order to make the game safe for everyone.

Activity Level The level appears only when the activity level of the game is mixed (i.e., low to moderate or moderate to high). Otherwise, the activity level of the game can be determined by the chapter in which it is included or can be found in the games finder.

Lead-Ins Lead-ins are games that work well when played before this game.

Number of Players The number of players is not often included as a category. That's because "the more the merrier" is almost always true. When it isn't, this heading appears, and we specify what you need to know. Otherwise, just remember that although a good general rule is to have one player for each panel of the parachute, fewer players can easily spread out around the parachute, and a couple of extra players can always squeeze in. Things start to get crowded when 40 players squeeze around a 24-foot (7.3-meter) parachute.

Developmental Skills   Skills, including social, personal behavior, perceptual, and basic motor skills, are fundamental to parachute games. We list these skills as primary or secondary, depending on their importance in a particular game. See chapter 3 for more detailed information about developmental skills.

No special motor skills are needed for any game; in fact, the games help develop some motor skills.

Additional Equipment   Extra equipment is required for some of the games. Items such as foam balls or Frisbees are noted here.

Duration of Game   The game should last as long as people are having fun. As a general guideline, most games last about five minutes. This category appears only when there are special considerations to be made for the length of the game. Remember that arms get tired when participants play a game such as Popcorn for longer than a few minutes. On the other hand, certain games such as Cat and Mouse have rounds in which only a few players have active roles. In these cases we recommend having enough time so that everyone gets a chance to play one of these roles.

Appropriate Ages   The majority of games are for all ages. We note the few exceptions.

When to Play   This is a tip on the best placement for a game in the context of a play session: beginning, middle, or ending activity.

Where to Play   This tip describes the optimal game space. You can play most parachute games almost anywhere. Of course, you'll need high ceilings when playing indoors. A few games require certain playing conditions; in such cases this category appears with any special considerations. For example, Parachute Ride and Alligator work best on a smooth, hardwood floor.

Follow-Ups   This list includes the games that work well after playing this particular game.

Variations   These are some ideas on how to take the game you just learned and make some changes to create a new game. This is our sneaky way of sharing more games with you while not adding more pages and increasing the cost of the book. Don't think that you need to play all the different variations of a game in one play session. One version will do fine. You can always play a different version in a future play session.

Teaching Tips   These tips are our way to pass along insights about the game and the way players may act during the game. These tips are based on our years of playing these games with many different types of groups in many different settings. These tips aren't part of the rules; you don't need to know them to be able to play the game. It is our hope that sharing these tips will make it easier and more fun for you and your players.

Here are three sample play sessions that have worked well for us. You might want to start out with these groupings, but the longer you play, the more you'll develop your own way of doing things and your own favorite game combinations. Don't be limited by our experience. Go out there—play, express yourself, and have a good time!

Sample Play Session 1

1. Wave Machine
2. Mushroom
3. Jumbo Mushroom
4. Igloo
5. Rocking Chair
6. Heartbeat
7. Racing Heartbeat
8. Cat and Mouse
9. Climb the Mountain
10. Drag Race

Sample Play Session 2

1. Free Play
2. Merry-Go-Round
3. World Record Merry-Go-Round
4. Snake Tag
5. Shark
6. Centipede
7. Cover Up
8. Circular Tug
9. Group Balance
10. Turnover

Sample Play Session 3

1. Popcorn
2. Big Bang
3. Gophers
4. Circular Sit-Ups
5. Ostrich
6. Blow Up
7. Cop and Robber
8. Ghost Rider
9. Turnover
10. It's in the Bag

Low-Activity
Parachute Games

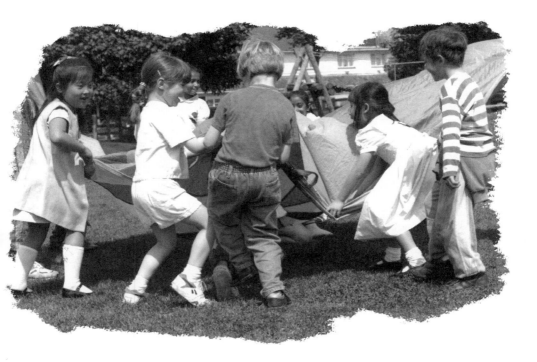

Name	Page number	When to play	Included on DVD
Big Bang	53	Middle	(disc)
Blow Up	54	Middle	(disc)
Cover Up	55	Middle	
Drag Race	56	Ending	(disc)
Floating Mushroom	57	Middle	
Free Play	59	Beginning	(disc)
Group Balance	61	Ending	(disc)
Igloo	62	Middle	(disc)
Interlocking Gears	63	Middle	
Jumbo Mushroom	65	Beginning	(disc)
Mushroom	66	Beginning	(disc)
Ostrich	68	Middle	(disc)
Over Under	69	Middle	
Parachute Golf	70	Middle	
Parachute Pass	71	Ending	
Parachute Ride	72	Ending	
Rabbit and Hound	74	Middle	
Rocking Chair	76	Middle	(disc)
Sculpture	77	Middle	
Swooping Cloud	78	Middle	
Turnover	80	Ending	(disc)
Wave Wall	81	Middle	
Who's Peeking?	82	Middle	

Here are 23 games that give you a chance to rest and play at the same time. Even people who have limited mobility can play these games. You can also use these games with any group when you want to keep things low key or when you want to take a breather after you've worn yourselves out with high-activity games.

Big Bang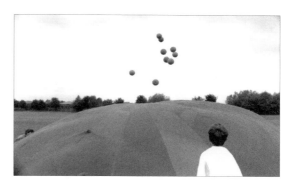

Have everyone spread the parachute on the ground and then place all the balls in the middle. "One, two, three, lift!" The players lift the parachute as quickly as possible to shoulder level and then snap it down. The effect is that the balls fly off the parachute. Congratulations—you have just demonstrated the big bang theory of how the universe began with one giant explosion.

For a little variety, try this game with one large ball instead of many little balls.

Lead-Ins   Popcorn, Floating Mushroom, Heartbeat, Igloo, other mushroom games.

Developmental Skills   Primary—cooperation; Secondary—self-control, reaction, strength.

Additional Equipment   Foam balls or other light, soft objects.

Duration of Game   Repeating this game numerous times takes about three minutes.

Appropriate Ages   Players under age 6 might have trouble lifting a large parachute.

When to Play   Middle.

Follow-Ups   Ghost Rider, Ball Surfing, Popcorn, Housekeeping, Popovers, Parachute Golf.

Variations   You can easily turn this into a fun, mildly competitive game by creating two opposing teams: the tossers and the catchers. The tossers hold on to the edge of the parachute while the catchers form a wider circle away from the parachute. The catchers try to catch as many balls as they can before the balls touch the ground. Catchers earn one point for each ball they catch.

Teaching Tips   If you have all of the taller, stronger players clumped together along one arc of the parachute, you will tend to have most of the balls fly off over the heads of the shorter players. You can ensure a more random dispersal of the balls by distributing your tall and short players evenly around the parachute.

Blow Up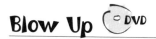

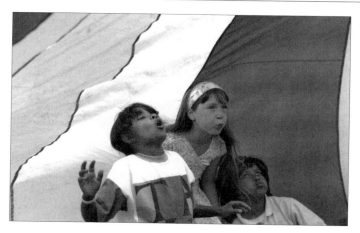

Blow Up can be considered a continuation of Ostrich; the object of Blow Up is to keep the parachute inflated. It takes a concerted effort with all the players using just their lungs and breath to keep the parachute up as long as possible. Don't be disheartened; the parachute settles to the ground eventually. By the way, this is great practice for blowing out birthday candles.

Lead-Ins   Ostrich, Who's Peeking?

Developmental Skills   Primary—cooperation; Secondary—spontaneity.

Duration of Game   It's a miracle if this lasts more than a minute.

When to Play   Middle.

Where to Play   Indoor space needs a high ceiling with protected lights.

Follow-Ups   Any game, especially moderate- or high-activity ones.

Variations   A goofy variation of this game is Vacuum. Instead of trying to keep the parachute inflated, everyone tries to deflate the parachute as quickly as possible by inhaling as strongly as they can.

Teaching Tips   It should come as no surprise that even the strongest-lunged group of nonsmokers can't really keep a parachute inflated. It's pretty fun to watch people try, though.

Cover Up

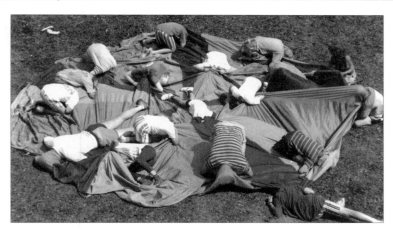

Have everyone lie down on her or his own section of a loosely laid-out parachute. The goal of this game is to see if all the players can find enough spare fabric at the same time to tuck themselves in. You can vary the activity by calling out specific body parts to wrap.

Lead-Ins   Centipede, Raceway, Flying Parachute, Treasure Hunt, Shark.

Developmental Skills   Secondary—problem solving, creativity, spontaneity, self-control.

Duration of Game   Only a few minutes.

When to Play   Middle.

Follow-Ups   Sculpture, Jellyfish Jaunt, Dodge 'Em, Top of the Pops, Rocking Chair.

Variations   After everyone is covered up comfortably, you can play some simultaneous gentle games of Tug-of-War. Have all the players pretend that they are sleeping and that they are accidentally pulling the covers over themselves as they roll in their sleep. The fun comes when two or more people end up trying to pull the same part of the parachute over themselves.

Teaching Tips   Although it is not required, a slight amount of touching may be involved in this game. Depending on the group, you may want to make sure that there is enough space on the parachute so that all the players have an ample amount of chute to cover themselves without having to be in close contact with other players. We recommend no more than about 20 players for a parachute with a 30-foot (9.1-meter) diameter. A chute with a 20-foot (6.1-meter) diameter works well with about 16 players. Of course, these numbers vary, depending on the size of your players.

Drag Race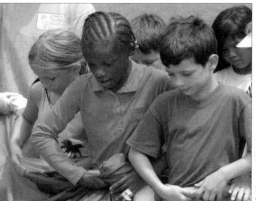

When you are finished playing with the parachute, don't just tell people you are through and get stuck packing up the chute alone. Instead, coax the players into helping you roll up the parachute.

The game is called Drag Race. It's easy to play, it's fun, and it quickly reduces the parachute into a nice, small bundle. Everyone is a drag racer. The object is to be the first drag racer to the middle of the parachute. Players get there by rolling the parachute up with their hands. Sound effects help. "Racers, start your engines. And they're off. Vroom!"

© Human Kinetics

Safety Tips   As players get closer to the middle, there is bound to be physical contact. Simply remind them not to hurt other racers.

Lead-Ins   Parachute Ride, Cover Up, I Dare Ya, any moderate or active game.

Developmental Skills   Primary—reaction; Secondary—self-control, skillfulness, coordination.

Duration of Game   About one minute.

When to Play   A perfect ending game.

Follow-Ups   It's in the Bag, Parachute Ride.

Variations   You can change the mood of the game by scoring players on how tightly they can roll up the parachute, rather than on how quickly. Of course, you should explain in advance that you are going to walk around and inspect the parachute to see how tightly each of the players has rolled up her or his section. It might be appropriate to give out a "White Knuckle" award to the players who are particularly tight rollers.

Teaching Tips   If your play session has been exuberant, the players may play an extreme version of Drag Race, complete with wheelies and stock-car crashes. That's okay. We have noticed that players may sometimes bump into each other as they race to the center, but these collisions are low speed. We have also found that this is an excellent way for players to burn off some of that excess energy.

Floating Mushroom

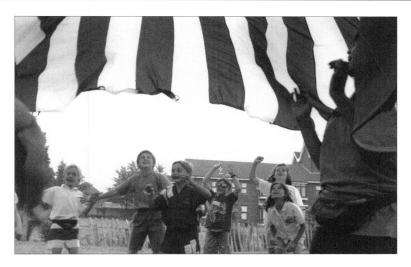

Floating Mushroom starts the same as Mushroom, but this time the players lift the parachute over their heads. When the leader gives a predetermined signal—such as "Now!" or "Let go!" or "Fungus Fly Free!"—everyone releases, or at least tries to release, the parachute simultaneously. (It's fun to caution the players that if everyone lets go of the parachute at exactly the same time, it just might keep on floating all the way up to the sky.)

Safety Tips   Encourage players to simply watch the parachute until it is all the way down. Children often have the desire to run into the parachute as it descends, which can be a lot of fun—until they run into each other at full speed.

Lead-Ins   Mushroom, Jumbo Mushroom, Big Bang, Climb the Mountain, Heartbeat.

Developmental Skills   Primary—cooperation, reaction; Secondary—verbal contact, adaptability, self-control, visual ability, strength.

Duration of Game   This game can be repeated a few times but is still over in minutes.

Appropriate Ages   6 years or over. Very young children (under 6 years) have trouble letting go together.

When to Play   Middle.

Where to Play   Indoor space should have a high ceiling.

Follow-Ups   Jell-O, Sculpture, Dodge 'Em, Centipede, any active game.

Variations   This variation of the game takes a lot of coordination. Players pretend they are at a sporting event and try to create a continuous, circular wave with the parachute. The players lift the chute up very slowly and then bring it down slowly, over and over. One person lets go. After her, the player to her right then lets go. Players continue letting go in sequence, all the while slowly raising and lowering the parachute. After five people have let go of the parachute, the first player regrabs the edge she was originally holding.

Players continue letting go and regrabbing the parachute, all the while maintaining a moving gap of five players who are not holding on to the chute. This gap is the wave of the parachute going around the stadium.

How many circuits can you send around the stadium before the wave breaks up on the shore?

Teaching Tips   This game is really a secret form of team building. The best Floating Mushrooms are achieved when everyone lets go of the parachute at exactly the same time. Taking into account barometric pressure and wind conditions, you can judge a well-synchronized team by how high the parachute floats.

Free Play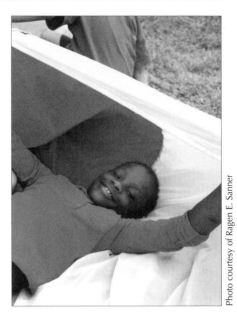

This parachute game may be obvious, but we are mentioning it to cover all bases. Very often people like to play with the parachute without any set game. Just put the parachute out and let the players experiment. It's fun to see what can happen.

Safety Tips We recommend that someone continue to watch over the activity, even though he or she is doing so passively. There are a couple of reasons for this. We would not want to see a claustrophobic player trapped in a seemingly hopeless tangle of parachute. Sometimes kids think covering someone else is a great game and they don't realize that it looks like more fun from the outside than from the inside.

Tossing someone up can be fun but can also be very dangerous. Actually, the tossing up part is always fun. It's the sudden stop if someone hits the ground that can be dangerous. Remember that army-surplus parachutes are no longer strong enough to stop someone from falling. That's why they are surplus!

Specially made play parachutes were never designed to stop people from falling. In addition, no matter how strong the parachute was the last time you used it, chances are that other people have used it since then, and it may be a parachute just waiting for a rip. We don't want to scare you, but we also want to make sure that no one gets hurt.

Lead-Ins Wave Rolling, Gophers, Jell-O, Cover Up, Merry-Go-Round.

Developmental Skills Primary—cooperation, problem solving, tactile contact, creativity, spontaneity, crawling; Secondary—adaptability, visual ability, balancing.

Additional Equipment Possibly foam balls to place under the parachute.

When to Play Beginning.

Follow-Ups Waves Overhead, I Dare Ya, Cop and Robber, Merry-Go-Round.

Photo courtesy of Ragen E. Sanner

Variations   This isn't actually a variation on Free Play. We are just sneaking this game in here because we like it.

It takes a little bit of preparation, but a nice game to play with a parachute is Concentration. Spread out the parachute loosely on the ground. You want to lay out the chute so that there is plenty of spare fabric to hide the treasures.

Place some objects randomly on the top of the chute, and cover them up with surplus material. Ask the players to slowly walk around and uncover various parts of the chute to temporarily reveal the objects that are hidden underneath. They should cover the objects back up after they have seen what treasure lies hidden under that section.

Concentration then becomes a memory game as you ask the players what objects were hidden under a certain section of the parachute.

Teaching Tips   In our experience Free Play with a parachute usually ends up being a great opportunity for some fun group wrestling. Kids frequently use the parachute as an excuse to crash into each other. That's fine, as long as they are low-speed crashes. Don't let people get a long, running start and then crash into other players. The thin fabric of the parachute doesn't offer any type of padding.

Group Balance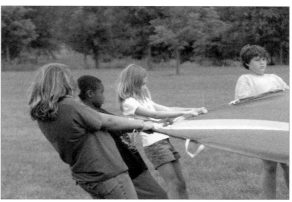

Make sure all the players have a good grip on the parachute, and then tell everyone to lean back slowly at the same time. Remember to make sure that the players roll up the edge several times with their fingers tucked in under the roll before leaning.

The parachute gets tighter and tighter, but a good strong parachute can support this type of evenly distributed tension. If everyone works together, all the players should be able to lean back quite far without losing their balance. If not, you get to find out which side of the parachute weighs the most! Oof!

For an added challenge, ask participants to turn their backs to the parachute, reach behind themselves for a grip, and then try to balance outward.

Safety Tips   Should be played on a soft surface such as grass or mats, especially if players are worried about falling.

Lead-Ins   Circular Sit-Ups, Merry-Go-Round, Dodge 'Em, Shark, Wave Wall.

Developmental Skills   Primary—cooperation, trust, verbal contact, balancing; Secondary—adaptability, self-control, visual ability.

Duration of Game   Likely only to last a few minutes.

When to Play   Ending.

Follow-Ups   Circular Tug, Ball Surfing, Ghost Rider, Liftoff, Drag Race.

Variations   See if your particular parachute favors a right-hand or a left-hand grip. Ask everyone to hold onto the parachute using just the right hand. Note how well they can balance as a group. Have them switch to their left hands. Was the balance the same, better, not as balanced?

You can also vary the game by having all of the players stand with their feet in various positions: shoulder-length apart, right next to each other, or really wide apart.

Teaching Tips   Don't be afraid to ask people to switch positions around the chute, if the group is in the mood to explore the subtleties of game.

Igloo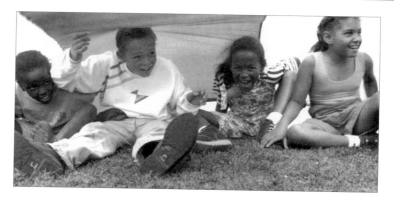

Players lift the parachute up into a giant mushroom, take a couple of steps in, and bring the parachute down behind them with everyone inside the chute sitting on the edge. You have just built the warmest igloo in the world. Not only does it look great from the outside, but from the inside it's also a wonderful place for telling secrets or playing the classic game of Telephone. And when it's time to get out, "The last one out is a turnip!"

Lead-Ins   Jumbo Mushroom, Heartbeat, other mushroom games.

Developmental Skills   Primary—cooperation, adaptability, skillfulness, coordination; Secondary—verbal contact, self-control, visual ability.

When to Play   Middle.

Follow-Ups   Rocking Chair, Blow Up, Centipede, Waves Overhead.

Variations   Try having people gently lie down, with all heads pointing to the inside of the circle. Make sure that everyone moves slowly and that no noggins are conked.

All the players point their feet straight up and try to tuck the parachute under their bums in a sort of Reverse Igloo.

Teaching Tips   This is a great game to play on a windy day. Being inside of an Igloo provides a natural windbreak. It also creates a sense of intimacy for the players under the chute, even when there are lots of other things happening on the field.

On a cold, windy day we have used the Igloo format to play a host of other games. Without the parachute, it would have been too cold to play these games.

Which games would be good to play under a parachute on a cold, windy day? Just about any game that involves people sitting in a circle makes for a great game.

Interlocking Gears

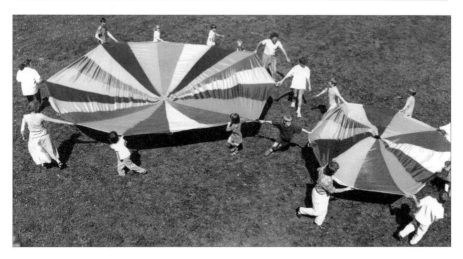

This game requires two parachutes. Place the two parachutes side by side so that they are almost touching. Both groups walk in a circle as in the Merry-Go-Round game. When players reach the point where the two parachutes meet, they grab ahold of the other parachute, let go of the one they were holding, and join the other circle. This means that people are walking in a giant figure-eight pattern (one circle rotates clockwise, the other counterclockwise). It takes timing and coordination between the two groups but eventually it goes like clockwork. After a while, have players reverse directions.

Lead-Ins Flying Parachute, Wave Rolling, Parachute Golf, any other high-activity game.

Number of Players 12 or more.

Developmental Skills Primary—walking, cooperation; Secondary—self-control, visual ability, verbal contact.

Additional Equipment Second parachute.

When to Play Middle.

Where to Play You need enough room to spread out two parachutes, plus a bit more.

Follow-Ups Parachute Volleyball, Sculpture, Merry-Go-Round, Missile Launch.

Variations Suggest that players can, at the critical moment, choose to switch to the other parachute or decide to stay with their home parachute. How will one player's decision affect the next player? How many teeth can the group load onto one parachute? How few teeth can a parachute have, before its gear winds down?

You could also try having gears (players) switch directions when called on to do so.

Teaching Tips Interlocking Gears may take a bit of trial and error before groups meet with success. That's okay. When the game is presented in a supportive, motivating way, it's a great feeling for the group to struggle a bit at the beginning and then break through into playing the game fluidly.

Jumbo Mushroom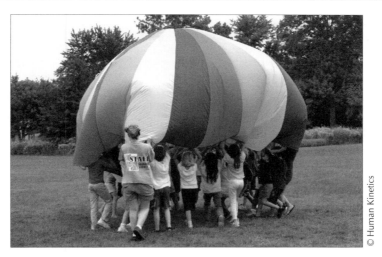

This game is similar to Mushroom, but this time as you lift the parachute, ask everyone to walk in a step or two. This makes the mushroom grow even bigger. Repeat the game with everyone taking an additional step. Each round makes the mushroom bigger, and eventually everyone meets in the middle.

Safety Tips   Have everyone slowly count out loud and step into the center together so that there are no high-speed collisions.

Lead-Ins   Mushroom, Heartbeat, Floating Mushroom, any more active game.

Developmental Skills   Primary—cooperation, adaptability; Secondary— verbal contact, self-control, visual ability, strength, walking.

When to Play   Beginning.

Where to Play   Requires a tall ceiling if played indoors.

Follow-Ups   Moderate- or high-activity game, Floating Mushroom, other mushroom games.

Variations   Keeping in mind that safety is the primary concern, have the group try different rhythms when making Jumbo Mushrooms. Try having everyone gradually speed up as they walk into the center. How about if they all try to move together as slowly as possible?

Teaching Tips   Making Jumbo Mushrooms is a great way to attract attention to the parachute and your play group. If you are playing in a public area, expect people to come over and ask what is going on.

Mushroom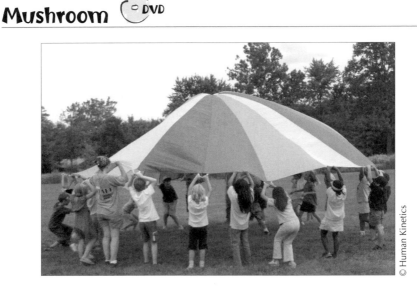

Here is something that involves teamwork, is not too hard, and looks beautiful. Everyone kneels down and holds the parachute taut on the ground. On the same count everyone stands up, lifting the parachute high up over their heads. A giant mushroom is formed. Have the players stand still and watch as the parachute slowly settles back down to the ground.

Having a hard time getting everyone to begin on the same count? One way to get people to lift the parachute together is on the universal word "Mushroom." Calling out preliminary vegetables such as "Broccoli" or "Asparagus" builds up the suspense.

Lead-Ins   Wave Machine, Free Play, popcorn games, any high-activity games.

Developmental Skills   Primary—cooperation, adaptability; Secondary—verbal contact, self-control, visual ability, strength.

When to Play   Beginning.

Where to Play   Requires a tall ceiling if played indoors.

Follow-Ups   Jumbo Mushroom, Floating Mushroom, or a moderate- or high-activity game.

Variations   Several variations on Mushrooms are already mentioned. See Floating Mushroom (page 57) and Jumbo Mushroom (page 65) for descriptions of these games. You can use a basic Mushroom to help your players learn to identify different body parts. As the mushroom growers lift up the parachute, call out directions involving different parts of the body. Here are some ideas:

"Grow a Mushroom with just your left hand." "Stand on your right leg." "Tilt your head to the left."

A more active version of Mushroom is called Searching for Truffles. In this game players are asked to leave their positions on the parachute to look for truffles and find a new spot around the chute. Someone calls out various categories of truffle hunters. The chosen categories have to switch positions. The difference between this game and Racing Heartbeat (page 138) is that the chosen players exchange positions on the outside of the parachute, instead of underneath the chute.

Teaching Tips When playing Searching for Truffles, make sure that the categories leave a fair amount of people around the perimeter of the parachute. A category such as "Everyone who is wearing the color blue" usually ensures that at least half of the group will let go of the parachute to look for truffles.

Ostrich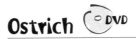

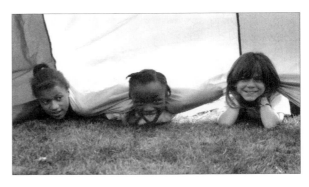

Here's a great game that looks as funny from the inside as it does from the outside. Everyone hoists the parachute and takes two steps in to form a Jumbo Mushroom. While the mushroom is descending, players get down on their bellies or knees, poke their heads under the parachute, and pull the parachute down around their shoulders. The view from the inside is a ring of disembodied smiling faces all looking at each other as the parachute slowly settles to the ground. Don't even think about what you look like to the people on the outside. It's best to pretend you are invisible to everyone but fellow ostriches.

Vary the game by reversing the process: bodies under the parachute and heads out.

Lead-Ins   Circular Tug, Climb the Mountain, any other moderate- or high-activity game.

Developmental Skills   Primary—cooperation; Secondary—self-control, skillfulness, coordination.

Duration of Game   This game will likely last only a minute or two.

When to Play   Middle.

Where to Play   Not on dirt, concrete, or blacktop.

Follow-Ups   Cat and Mouse, Circular Sit-Ups, Cover Up.

Variations   Have the ostriches stay still and pass the parachute over their necks to their neighbors. See how far along the circle you can all pass the parachute before the middle touches the ground.

Teaching Tips   You may want to be aware of other people who are around the parachute and are not part of the group. If you think that there are bored people in the area who tend toward aggressive behavior or who may act up, you may not want to have your players play Ostrich. When the players, or ostriches, cannot see the people outside the parachute and their bodies are extended outside the parachute, the players are vulnerable to the taunts or mischief of others.

Over Under

Want to turn the parachute over quickly? Make a mushroom and have one side let go of the parachute. Then have both sides trade positions as fast as possible. Watch out for the parachute.

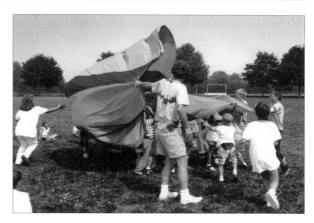

Lead-Ins Turnover, Floating Mushroom, Heartbeat, any Mushroom game.

Developmental Skills Primary—verbal contact, visual ability; Secondary—cooperation, adaptability, walking, self-control, reaction.

Appropriate Ages 6 and over.

When to Play Middle.

Follow-Ups Flying Parachute, Circular Tug, Jell-O, Sculpture.

Variations Give extra points if players change sides by following specific suggestions. For example, have everyone on the team that lets go circle around the outside of the parachute in a counterclockwise direction. Or have players switch sides by passing between the players who remain holding on to the chute.

Teaching Tips Low-speed collisions between players are a lot more fun than high-speed collisions. Players can have safe, fun, low-speed collisions over and over. Fortunately, the relatively small space defined by the perimeter of the parachute acts as a built-in governor, which limits the speed at which players can crash into each other. Don't feel shy about reminding people to slow down if you see that they are getting a bit too excited.

Parachute Golf

If your parachute has a hole in the middle, you can play a round of Parachute Golf. It takes quite a bit of teamwork to get the ball to roll through the hole. We would guess about a par 47.

For young children, a smaller ball makes it easier to get a hole in one.

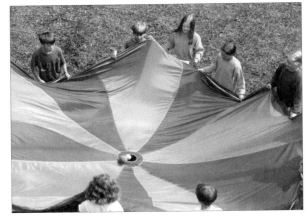

Lead-Ins Ball Surfing, Ghost Rider, Popovers, Making Waves, Popcorn.

Developmental Skills Primary—cooperation; Secondary—verbal contact, adaptability, visual ability, strength.

Additional Equipment A ball small enough to go through the hole in the parachute.

Duration of Game Length of game may vary from 5 to 10 minutes.

When to Play Middle.

Follow-Ups Housekeeping, Missile Launch, Rabbit and Hound, Snake Tag.

Variations You may also play a competitive version of this game. Create two teams—the golfers and the spoilers—by alternating players around the parachute. The golfers are evenly interspersed among the spoilers. Golfers try to get the ball in the hole. Spoilers try to keep the ball out of the hole.

You may want to have timed rounds. Have the teams switch roles after 60 seconds. Was one team a particularly good spoiler?

Teaching Tips This game takes a surprising amount of cooperation and group concentration. Young players may occasionally find it frustrating to get the ball to roll into the hole. You can make it easier for younger players by "choking up" on the parachute. Have everyone roll the lip of the parachute several turns so the diameter of the chute becomes shorter. A smaller parachute gives more control to the players, especially shorter players.

Parachute Pass

In this game all the players stand still and pass a bit of the parachute to their neighbor. The parachute is passed from hand to hand, but the players are not allowed to cross their arms. One hand should be holding on at all times. The object is to try to pass faster than you receive. You are doing a good job if

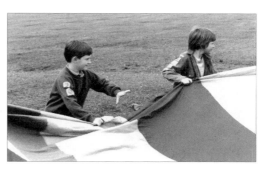

there is a lot of loosely draped parachute by the neighbor to whom you are passing but on your other side the parachute is tight.

Lead-Ins Group Balance, Circular Tug, any mushroom, popcorn, or more active game.

Developmental Skills Primary—reaction; Secondary—self-control, skillfulness and coordination, tactile contact, adaptability, spontaneity, visual ability.

Duration of Game One to two minutes.

When to Play Ending.

Follow-Ups Drag Race, It's in the Bag, Group Balance, Circular Sit-Ups.

Variations A fun variation of this game is to have all of the players interlock their arms with the arms of their neighbors. Everyone places his or her left arm over the right arm of the player to his or her left. Now passing the parachute becomes a cooperative effort instead of a competitive one.

Teaching Tips Even though all of the players are standing still, this game can still become quite frantic. Be sure that all of the players maintain their sense of personal boundaries. In the excitement of play, some players may overreach as they pass the parachute and may crowd into the space of another player.

Parachute Ride

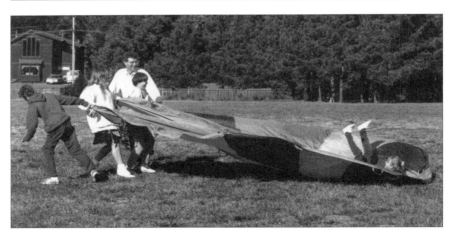

Parachutes don't always have to be round or fully extended in order for players to have fun with them. Not many people can participate in a parachute ride at any one time, but for the lucky one or two who do get a lift, it's a memorable trip.

Designate one or two players to lie down on top of the parachute, near the center. The other players all grab ahold of an edge on either side of the parachute. The group then goes for a walk, turning the parachute into a giant sled or travois for the riders.

Safety Tips   Make sure that the team members pulling the parachute don't go over any harmful surfaces, such as rocks or holes.

Lead-Ins   Climb the Mountain, Merry-Go-Round, I Dare Ya, Jell-O.

Number of Players   Fewer than 12.

Developmental Skills   Primary—strength; Secondary—visual ability, walking, balancing, creativity, spontaneity.

When to Play   Ending.

Where to Play   Best on a slippery surface.

Follow-Ups   Free Play, Liftoff, Drag Race, It's in the Bag.

Variations   Instead of dragging people around on top of the parachute, try rolling them gently off of the chute. A Rollover begins with one player lying down just to one side of the center of the chute. Players around the far edge of the parachute walk around the player who is lying down so that she is completely covered by the chute. Picture a giant, human-filled taco.

At this point the players holding the top half of the chute gently pull on the parachute. The goal is to nudge and roll the person off of the parachute. Make sure the majority of the pull of the parachute is perpendicular to the direction in which the person is lying down. Imagine a log rolling out of the chute, and you have the idea.

Teaching Tips   Please be aware of the surface on which you are playing. We only recommend taking people for parachute rides on gym floors or on smooth, even grass. Asphalt doesn't work too well. Even on grass, you may not want to play this particular game if you are concerned about grass stains on your parachute. You can protect your parachute by placing a large piece of cardboard between the parachute and the ground.

Rabbit and Hound

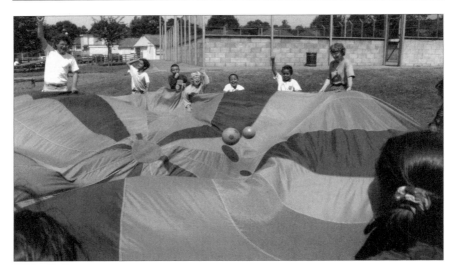

Throw two unlike balls on top of the parachute. Different sizes and different colors work well. Two teams are trying to control the destiny of the two balls. One ball is the hound, and the other is the rabbit. One team tries to help the hound catch the rabbit while the other team is trying to help the rabbit get away.

The teams can be divided several different ways, and each arrangement results in different team strategies. You can draw an imaginary line down the middle of the parachute to divide the teams, or you can create teams that consist of every other person around the edge. An interesting variation might be dividing the parachute into quarters and having the two opposing quadrants work together as a team.

Lead-Ins   Ball Surfing, Housekeeping, Parachute Basketball, any ball games.

Developmental Skills   Primary—cooperation, visual ability, strength; Secondary—problem solving, verbal contact, adaptability, self-control, reaction, endurance.

Additional Equipment   Two different types or colors of balls; a basketball and a volleyball work well.

Duration of Game   This game could end quickly, and roles could be reversed and played again for another round. In any case, the game usually ends in two to three minutes.

When to Play   Middle.

Follow-Ups   Gophers, Missile Launch, Parachute Golf, Parachute Volley-ball.

Variations   Modify the game by having two hounds chase one rabbit. Color-code the two hounds and you can divide the parachute into three teams: two hounds and a rabbit.

Or give one hound two different rabbits to catch.

Teaching Tips   This game involves a lot of continuous, strenuous shaking. You may want to play the game in short, timed rounds. If the rabbit can elude the hound for a full minute (or 30 seconds), the rabbit scores a point.

Rocking Chair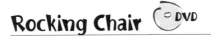

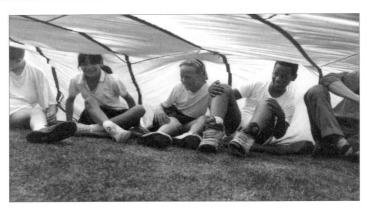

While the players are still inside an Igloo, they can make a giant Rocking Chair. Instead of rocking back and forth, this rocking chair tends to rock in a circular motion. Can you make it rock in a clockwise and then a counter-clockwise direction? Begin with small movements. Before too long, a group rhythm develops and then gets amplified.

Lead-Ins   Igloo, Centipede, Ostrich, any high-activity game.

Developmental Skills   Primary—cooperation, adaptability; Secondary—self-control, skillfulness, coordination.

When to Play   Middle.

Follow-Ups   Any moderate- or high-activity game.

Variations   You can try to create a seated Heartbeat by having everyone lean in and lean back at the same time.

Teaching Tips   Some players may only hold the parachute around their backs with their hands. Although that works somewhat, this game is more fun if all of the players are actually sitting on the edge of the parachute. Physically sitting on the chute makes for a nice, snug Rocking Chair.

Sculpture

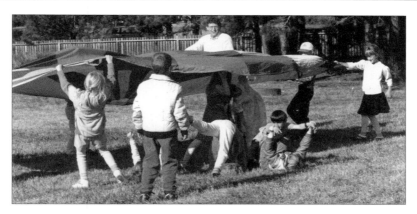

Ask three to six players to go underneath the parachute while everyone else makes a mushroom. The players in the middle form themselves into a living sculpture as the parachute settles down around them. Some go high, some go low, and all together they form a giant piece of modern art. Once the parachute descends, everyone can admire the wrapped artwork.

Finally, the sculpture is ready, and it's time to unveil the work of art. If you like, you can make a guessing game before the unveiling to see if people on the outside of the parachute can guess what the form is or who is making what shape.

Lead-Ins   I Dare Ya, Racing Heartbeat, Gophers, Flying Parachute, Merry-Go-Round.

Developmental Skills   Primary—cooperation, trust, problem solving, tactile contact, creativity, spontaneity, self-control; Secondary—adaptability, balancing, trust, verbal contact, visual ability, leaning.

When to Play   Middle.

Follow-Ups   Jellyfish Jaunt, World Record Merry-Go-Round, Pony Express, Raceway.

Variations   Before the unveiling you can ask everyone on the outside of the parachute to slowly walk up and touch one part of the sculpture with just the tip of one finger. After the unveiling, see if the pieces of the sculpture recognize who touched them.

Teaching Tips   Some players may try to define the Sculpture in greater detail by pulling the chute down tightly over the players underneath. If necessary, remind players to let the parachute fall gently over the Sculpture. Also, unless you specifically allow it, there is no touching of the Sculpture underneath the chute. This isn't a tactile museum exhibit.

Swooping Cloud

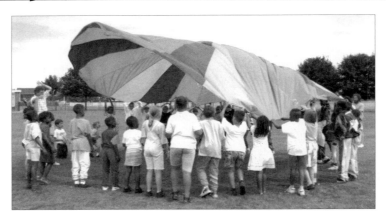

This game begins like the Floating Mushroom, but not everyone lets go at the same time. In fact, one side intentionally lets go after the other side. The parachute will then make a swooping cloud as it rises up on one side and comes right back down to the ground on the other side.

Lead-Ins   Floating Mushroom, Mushroom, Heartbeat, any mushroom game.

Developmental Skills   Primary—cooperation; Secondary—verbal contact, visual ability, reaction, strength.

Duration of Game   This is a very short game that can be repeated many times in just a few minutes.

When to Play   Middle.

Where to Play   Very low ceilings make this game difficult.

Follow-Ups   Over Under, Flying Parachute, any moderate- or high-activity game.

Variations   This variation is for really active players. If your group has a lot of energy, this will help them burn it up.

After the individual players let go of the parachute, they run around the outside to a space behind the "last-to-let-goers." It is a race to see if all the "initial releasers" can get to and stand behind the last-to-let-goers before the parachute settles down to the ground.

You can make this race against the parachute even more challenging by not letting all of the players know in advance who the last-to-let-goers are. All eyes are closed before the round begins. Walk around the outside of the parachute. Tap two or three players on the shoulder to let them know they will be the last-to-let-goers for the next round. All of the initial releasers must first look and determine the direction of the Swooping Cloud before they try to run behind the holders.

Teaching Tips   The more that everyone understands and carries out his or her role, the larger the effect of the Swooping Cloud. Make sure that all of the players know whether they are going to let go of the parachute or hold on to it.

If your group is sophisticated enough, you may even suggest that the players let go of the parachute in a more precise order, not just in two teams. The players on the opposite side of the last-to-let-goers will be the first two to let go of the chute. Players on both sides of the initial releasers hold on for just a bit longer before releasing the parachute. The idea is to begin with one side of the chute billowing up, and then most of the chute billows up before it swoops down again.

Turnover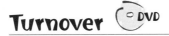

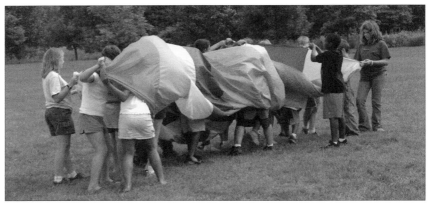

© Human Kinetics

Here's a group challenge. Can you turn the parachute over with no one letting go of the edge? It takes lots of teamwork and communication. Oh, and some trust and delicate footwork are helpful, too.

Lead-Ins   Over Under, Jellyfish Jaunt, Parachute Pass, Centipede, Circular Tug.

Developmental Skills   Primary—cooperation, verbal contact, tactile contact, adaptability, spontaneity; Secondary—problem solving, creativity, balancing.

When to Play   Ending.

Follow-Ups   Sculpture, Jell-O, Cop and Robber, Circular Sit-Ups.

Variations   Try to have the group turn the parachute over without moving their feet. In this variation people are temporarily allowed to let go of the parachute.

Teaching Tips   There's actually an extremely easy way to accomplish this group challenge. Designate two adjacent players as the gatekeepers. Have everyone else walk through this human gate in single or double file. The players standing next to the gatekeepers are the first to pass through the gate, with subsequent players determined by the perimeter of the collapsing parachute. Everyone slowly walks toward the gate to provide enough slack for the people to pass between the gatekeepers. The parachute will be quite limp as players pass through the gate. The task is complete when the two gatekeepers each pirouette to finish the turnover.

Don't let the players know about this method too soon, though. It's too much fun watching the confusion of everybody inching their way over the parachute simultaneously.

Wave Wall

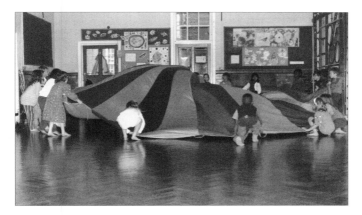

Hold the parachute still and have one small arc of people send a wave across the ocean to the other side. Did it get there? Can the people who received the wave pass on an even bigger one to another arc of the parachute? How big can these tidal waves get? What happens when two waves meet in the center?

Lead-Ins Swooping Cloud, Parachute Golf, Big Bang, any mushroom game.

Developmental Skills Primary—cooperation; Secondary—self-control, visual ability, strength, verbal contact, adaptability, reaction.

Duration of Game This game may last only two or three minutes.

When to Play Middle.

Follow-Ups Over Under, Popovers, Rabbit and Hound, Ghost Rider, Ball Surfing.

Variations Try placing a Frisbee, or some other light object that does not roll, on top of the parachute. Have the players work together to try to make small waves that surf the Frisbee over to a specific area of the chute.

Teaching Tips With guidance from the leader, this game can go from subtle ripples in a quiet pond to giant waves crashing on rocky shores.

Who's Peeking?

While you are play-
ing Ostrich or Igloo,
you can also play this
favorite game of ours.
We call it "Who's
Peeking?" The object
is to have all players
close their eyes and
then see who is peek-
ing. The best players
are the ones who
can catch the others
peeking without get-

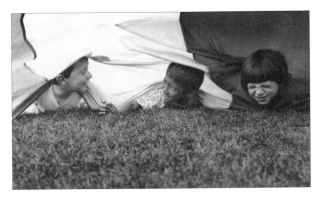

ting caught themselves. We saw that: you're peeking!

Lead-Ins   Ostrich, Igloo, Rocking Chair, Raceway.

Developmental Skills   Primary—cooperation, spontaneity, visual ability, reaction; Secondary—verbal contact, self-control, skillfulness and coordination.

Duration of Game   This game won't last longer than three minutes.

When to Play   Middle.

Follow-Ups   Wave Wall, Alligator, Parachute Pass, Over Under, any more
active game.

Variations   To make things more frantic, impose a time limit on the game.
Explain that everyone has just 10 (or 15) seconds to catch someone peeking.
    Another variation is to ask everyone to peek at the same time. This group
peek lasts only for an instant, with one quick, group opening of both eyes,
and then all eyes tightly shut again. Before the peek everyone chooses to
remove one shoe, two shoes, or no shoes. After the group peek, with eyes
shut players try to correctly state the status of their fellow players' shoes. If
having players remove and replace shoes is too complicated, suggest that
they hold one, two, or no hands on their shoulders.

Teaching Tips   Who's Peeking? is also a fun game to play when you are
inside of a giant Rocking Chair. There is a small risk of players caring too
much about this game. We have found that young players may occasionally
become upset if they are accused of peeking. We figure it's because of the
negative connotation of being accused of something one is not supposed to
be doing. Please remember to share the fact that this is just a goofy game,
and no one's reputation is being impugned.

Moderate-
Activity
Parachute Games

6

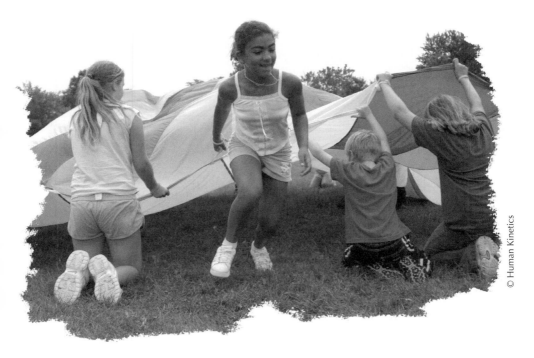

© Human Kinetics

Name	Page number	When to play	Included on DVD
Alligator	85	Middle	
Ball Surfing	87	Middle	
Centipede	89	Middle	⊙
Circular Sit-Ups	91	Middle	⊙
Circular Tug	93	Middle	⊙
Climb the Mountain	95	Ending	⊙
Cop and Robber	97	Middle	⊙
Dodge 'Em	99	Middle	
Ghost Rider	100	Middle	⊙
Gophers	102	Middle	⊙
Heartbeat	104	Beginning	⊙
It's in the Bag	105	Ending	⊙
Liftoff	107	Middle	
Missile Launch	109	Middle	
Parachute Basketball	111	Middle	
Parachute Volleyball	112	Middle	
Popovers	114	Middle	
Shark	116	Middle	⊙
Treasure Hunt	117	Middle	
Wave Machine	118	Beginning	⊙
Waves Overhead	119	Middle	

To help you vary the energy level of your play session, we include 21 games in this chapter that we consider moderately active.

Alligator

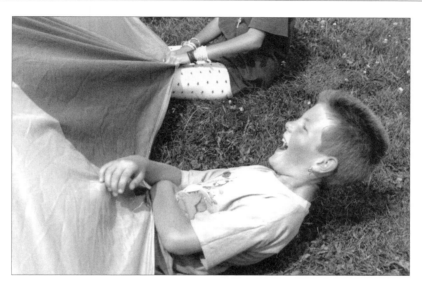

Alligator is a more moderate variation of the high-energy game, Shark. Instead of standing, all the players sit with their legs underneath the parachute, which has become a giant swamp. Very small waves help the swamp come alive.

Choose one player to be the alligator. The alligator crawls underneath the parachute to enter the swamp.

The exciting part of this game is when the alligator gets hungry. What hungry alligator could resist all those delicious legs floating under the edge of the swamp? Hungry alligators chomp onto another player by grabbing ahold of a leg, ankle, or foot with their hands. If you get bitten, you become the alligator; and the previous alligator joins the rest of the group. If someone does not want to be eaten by an alligator or has already been an alligator and wants to let others have a chance to chomp, that player should sit with legs crossed underneath himself or herself instead of under the parachute.

Instead of just biting unsuspecting players as in Shark, alligators can actually grab ahold of someone's leg and gently drag that player under the parachute and into the swamp. Watching a fellow wader go under makes quite an impression on the survivors at the swamp's edge.

In another version the players do not switch roles. Alligators create new alligators by biting waders and remain alligators until the end. The game is over when the swamp is full of alligators and no players are left to munch.

Safety Tips   Alligators who are too rough on waders may need a reminder that this is just for fun.

Lead-Ins   Group Balance, Raceway, Circular Sit-Ups, Ghost Rider, popcorn games.

Developmental Skills   Primary—cooperation, tactile contact, spontaneity, pantomime, crawling; Secondary—strength, leaning, verbal contact, adaptability, self-control.

When to Play   Middle.

Follow-Ups   Cat and Mouse, Cover Up, Missile Launch, Circular Tug, Ball Surfing.

Variations   If you think the players can handle the excitement of being pulled under quite rapidly, you can mention that alligators have been known to work in pairs. Two alligators working in tandem, each with one alligator mouth (hand) on an unsuspecting victim, make quite an impression. We're not sure which is more fun: being pulled under by a pair of alligators or watching the surprised look of someone else being pulled under.

Teaching Tips   We have found that different groups enjoy different levels of gore in this game. Squeamish alligator hunters may not enjoy this game and may choose to only dangle their feet in the swamp for light nips. More adventurous players may choose to build the tension by incorporating lots of alligator noises as they hunt.

Ball Surfing

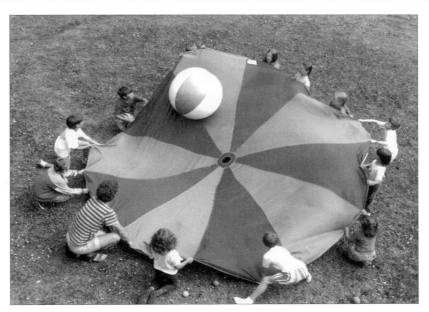

Place a large ball on top of the parachute and roll it around the edge. Players should lift the parachute just after the ball passes by. Timing is critical. If someone lifts up a section of the parachute too soon, the ball slows down and stops. If someone lifts a section too late, the ball either runs into the player or rolls off the parachute.

The smaller the ball, the greater the challenge. The larger the ball, the easier the game will be and the greater the effect. This game is even more fun with an Earthball.

Lead-Ins   Group Balance, Circular Tug, Dodge 'Em, Ghost Rider, popcorn games.

Developmental Skills   Primary—cooperation, visual ability, reaction; Secondary—adaptation, self-control, strength, verbal contact.

Additional Equipment   A large ball.

Appropriate Ages   This game will be a challenge for players younger than 6 years old.

When to Play   Middle.

Follow-Ups   Wave Wall, Merry-Go-Round, Parachute Volleyball, Cop and Robber.

Variations   If you have two smaller balls, and if the group is up for even more of a challenge, suggest that they try to keep two balls surfing around the parachute. The two balls should maintain their separation at opposite sides of the parachute as they both roll around. The action of raising and lowering the parachute becomes more precise, even as it occurs more frequently.

Teaching Tips   Look around the perimeter of the parachute and make sure that there aren't any gaps or huge size discrepancies between the players. A tall person's "arms down" may be a short person's "arms up." Remind the tall people to bend down extra low if they are next to shorter players.

Also, it takes some groups a bit of time to master the team coordination to actually get the ball surfing around the chute. The feeling of shared success after some failed initial attempts is pretty nice, though. We recommend that you not start this game unless you think you have enough time to let people experiment with it a bit.

Centipede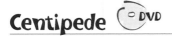

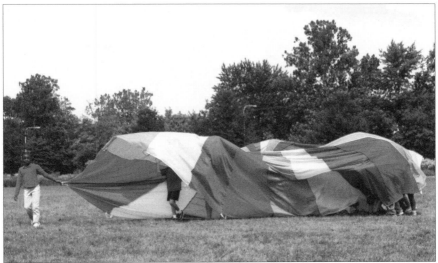

Photo courtesy of Ragen E. Sanner

Have you ever gone on a group hike? Here is a way to guarantee that there aren't any stragglers. All players help to lift the parachute up over their heads; then they all step underneath and let the parachute settle down over them. Once the parachute comfortably covers everyone, it is time to begin the walk. Watching the centipede is as much fun as being the centipede; you might want to divide the group into scientists and bugs and give everyone a turn to be on each side.

Safety Tips   The result looks like a very obese, undisciplined centipede. For this reason, it is good to appoint someone to be the "brain" of the centipede. The brain directs activities and avoids collisions. Curiously enough, this centipede's brain lives outside the parachute. Although this exterior brain baffles biologists, it makes for a safer game.

Activity Level   Low to moderate.

Lead-Ins   Blow Up, Waves Overhead, Racing Heartbeat, any game.

Developmental Skills   Primary—verbal contact; Secondary—cooperation, adaptability, spontaneity, visual ability, walking.

When to Play   Middle.

Where to Play   You will need some open space around the parachute for any type of decent walk.

Follow-Ups Jellyfish Jaunt, Flying Parachute, Cop and Robber, most any game.

Variations Instruct the centipede to go for a walk, and then see if it can find its way home to the exact starting point at which it began its journey.

Teaching Tips Depending on the terrain and the group, you may want to stress that this is a listening game; the exterior brain controls where the centipede walks. The guardian, or guardians, acting as the brain will see to it that the centipede doesn't inadvertently trample innocent bystanders and picnics.

Circular Sit-Ups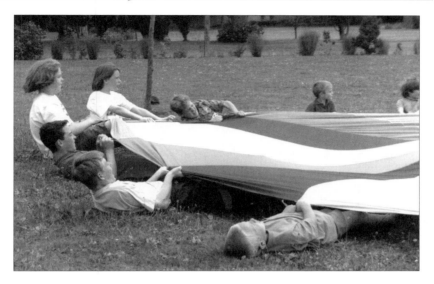

We find normal sit-ups a bit boring. We think it's easier, and certainly more fun, to perform one giant circular sit-up.

Have the players sit along the edge of the parachute with feet and legs underneath, holding on tightly to the edge of the parachute. One section starts to lean back while the opposite side leans forward. The two sides continue in this manner to create a seesaw effect. The whole group is doing sit-ups, sort of. For the moment players on the sides merely sway from side to side. That was just a warm up for Circular Sit-Ups.

The movement you need for circular sit-ups is more similar to the roundabout rocking motion of Rocking Chair than to the straight up-and-down motion of a traditional sit-up. If every player circles from the waist, the parachute will move accordingly. For the group to master this collective movement, you as leader may need to orchestrate the players a little. Point out which section of the parachute should be leaning back and then circling to the side until the players get the hang of it. Once the group has mastered both clockwise and counterclockwise sit-ups, try reversing directions without stopping.

Lead-Ins Igloo, Merry-Go-Round, World Record Merry-Go-Round, Dodge 'Em.

Developmental Skills Primary—cooperation; Secondary—adaptability, strength, self-control.

Duration of Game Players probably won't want to play for more than a minute or two.

When to Play Middle.

Follow-Ups Group Balance, Circular Tug, Ball Surfing, Alligator.

Variations Add some challenge to this game by suggesting that players hold on to the chute with only one hand instead of with both hands. Even more challenging is to have them constantly switch hands. Have them sit up holding the chute with one hand and sit back down holding on with the other hand.

Teaching Tips You can start this game very slowly. It might even be appropriate to suggest that people learn the basic Circular Sit-Up in slow motion. Once everyone has the basic idea, try speeding it up.

Circular Tug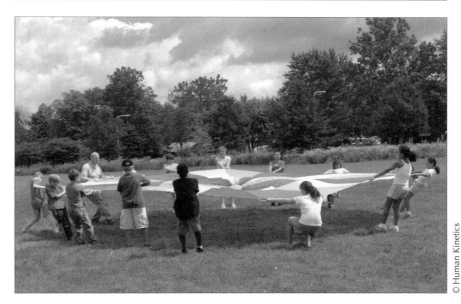

DVD

© Human Kinetics

This is an inverted version of Group Balance. Instead of everyone working together to stay balanced, the players compete in a circular tug-of-war. Everyone rolls up the edge of the parachute a few times and pulls straight back to see which side (or arc) of the parachute is the strongest. For those who like to see how they are doing, place a ball, Frisbee, or other marker on the ground underneath the middle of the parachute to start. Don't get pulled over the marker!

A challenging variation of this game is to ask participants to turn their back to the parachute, reach behind themselves for a grip, and then have a tug.

Safety Tips   Tugging games are safer, last longer, and are more fun if the players exert steady force. Consistent pulls are better than quick jerks. Also, make sure players don't have their fingers wrapped too tightly in the fold of the parachute's edge. You want the players to be able to get their fingers out quickly if they need to.

Lead-Ins   Group Balance; Alligator; any mushroom, popcorn, or low-activity game.

Number of Players   24 or fewer. This game sometimes ends with people falling down, so we don't like to overload the game with too many players. Make sure that the weight and strength of the players are evenly distributed and you can play with surprisingly few people.

Developmental Skills   Secondary—cooperation, adaptability, strength, verbal contact, self-control, spontaneity, visual ability, balancing.

Additional Equipment   A Frisbee or a ball as a marker.

Appropriate Ages   All ages can play, but make sure players of different ages and sizes are spread out evenly around the parachute.

When to Play   Middle.

Follow-Ups   Shark; Ball Surfing; Circular Sit-Ups; Merry-Go-Round; Jellyfish Jaunt; Ghost Rider; any mushroom, popcorn, or low-activity game.

Variations   A version of this game that uses the upper body instead of the waist includes having the players alternate between pulling their arms in and giving an arm's length of slack. Players on one side pull the parachute up to their chins while players on the other side extend their arms forward. Quickly reverse the motions to see how fast the group can move the taut chute back and forth. Of course, with a circle you have several options. You can move the parachute back and forth along the X- and Y-axes. With a bit more group coordination, the group can have the parachute circle in a clockwise or counterclockwise direction. This variation turns the parachute into a giant group rowing machine.

Teaching Tips   Scan the perimeter of the parachute to make sure that the sizes of the players are evenly distributed. Circular Tug is a bit lopsided if all the big players are concentrated along one arc of the chute.

Climb the Mountain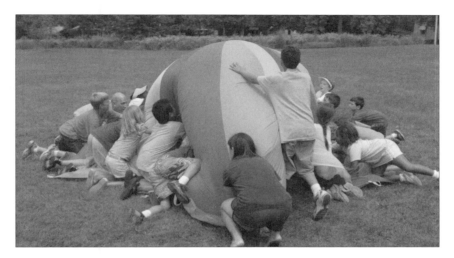

Players first make a giant mushroom. Then on a given verbal signal—such as "Down!"—they bring the parachute down quickly and hold the edge down with their knees. This traps the air underneath the parachute. Now players pretend to be mountain climbers and on their knees, try to scramble up the snowy mountain of cloth using just their arms.

Safety Tips   As enthusiastic climbers reach the middle, you may want to remind them to watch out for fellow climbers' heads on the other side of the mountain. Although all players stay on the same horizontal plane, the illusion is that the players are climbing up a mountain because the parachute gets smaller and smaller. Also, make it clear to players that they should not go under the parachute in this game.

Lead-Ins   Mushroom, Big Bang, Floating Mushroom, Wave Wall, Ostrich, any game.

Developmental Skills   Primary—cooperation, reaction, crawling; Secondary—verbal contact, tactile contact, visual ability.

Appropriate Ages   Between 6 and 60; younger and older players might find the game a bit too physical.

When to Play   Ending.

Where to Play   Best played on a soft surface.

Follow-Ups   Drag Race, Circular Sit-Ups, Group Balance, It's in the Bag, any low-activity game.

Variations   Instead of mountain climbers scaling a mountain, suggest that the players become squirrels and scamper up the tree as quickly as possible. Big, heavy, bears climb up trees much differently than light, frisky squirrels. Have the players demonstrate the difference between bears lumbering up a tree and squirrels scampering up. Or have players imitate snakes slithering up the tree.

Teaching Tips   The longer the parachute is supported by air, the more fun this game becomes. Try to have all of the players seal off the parachute by kneeling on the edge. This helps prevent the air from escaping.

Cop and Robber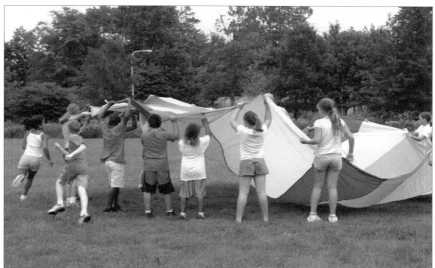

DVD

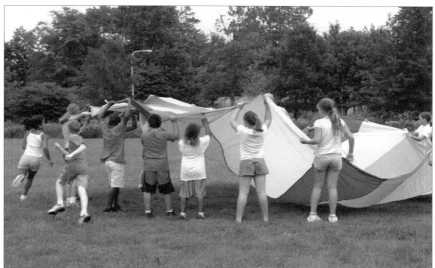

© Human Kinetics

"Stop! Thief!" And the chase is on. The robber makes a dash for her hideout. Her gang attempts to close ranks after her, thereby keeping the cop out. Actually, the robber can go underneath or outside the parachute while the cop tries to follow. The players around the parachute let the robber in or out but shift positions to get in the way and prevent the cop from following.

Justice is served when the robber gets caught. Then it's time to choose a new cop and a new robber. Later, try introducing two cops and two robbers.

Safety Tips   If the robbers around the parachute are too rough on the cop, you may need to ask them to give the long arm of the law a chance. After all, the chase is the fun part.

Lead-Ins   Shark, Flying Parachute, Pony Express, Waves Overhead, Popcorn.

Developmental Skills   Primary—cooperation, trust, adaptability, visual ability, reaction, speed, running; Secondary—problem solving, verbal contact, self-control, pantomime, leaning.

When to Play   Middle.

Follow-Ups   Alligator, Wave Rolling, Jellyfish Jaunt, Merry-Go-Round, Centipede.

Variations   Introduce the option of a role reversal into the game. When you yell, "Switch," the cop and the robber reverse roles.

The cop and the robber each may also take a break with the option to transfer their roles to any other players around the chute. Transfers are made with a simple tag and the pronouncement, "I deputize you!" or "You're on the lam!"

Teaching Tips   Things sure do get crowded when a posse of cops chases a gang of robbers. You can plan on collisions. To ensure that the ambulance doesn't show up, slow both sides of the law down to at least a fast walk, in which one foot has to touch the ground before the other foot is allowed to take a step.

Dodge 'Em

Here is a nice varia-
tion on that classic
old game of dodge-
ball. We use soft
foam balls instead
of playground balls
because the distance
is so much shorter
than in dodgeball
and foam is less
dangerous. A few
players go under the
parachute; everyone
else holds the para-

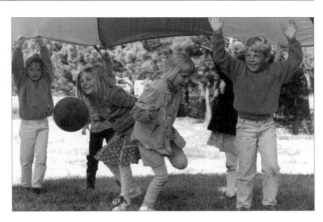

chute about head high. The added challenge is to have someone try to throw
the ball while holding on to the parachute with one hand and bending over
to see underneath the chute. The awkwardness in throwing is nicely balanced
by the dodger having to deal with an overhead parachute that restricts every
movement.

Lead-Ins   Alligator, Heartbeat, Ostrich, Missile Launch, any low- or high-
activity game.

Developmental Skills   Primary—adaptability, spontaneity, visual ability,
crawling, throwing and catching; Secondary—cooperation, problem solving, self-control, verbal contact, pantomime, skillfulness and coordination,
jumping.

Additional Equipment   One or two foam balls, perhaps more for younger
children.

When to Play   Middle.

Follow-Ups   Treasure Hunt, Waves Overhead, Who's Peeking?, Parachute
Basketball.

Variations   Our motto is "The more chaos, the more fun." Try playing Dodge
'Em with two foam balls instead of just one. Did we mention that hitting a
player with a ball results in the thrower and the dodger changing positions?
It does and they do, if you choose.

Teaching Tips   We've noticed that having lots of players under the chute at
one time increases the opportunity for a dodger to avoid being hit by the ball.
Remind everyone to play fairly. At an extreme, dodgers who can't seem to feel
being hit by the ball can sit out for a few minutes of sensitivity training.

Ghost Rider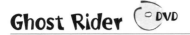

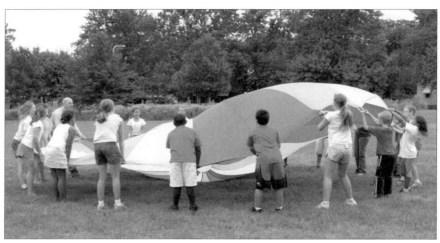

© Human Kinetics

A long time ago, there lived a daredevil motorcycle rider. He loved to ride his motorcycle faster and faster and jump over taller and taller obstacles. One day he and his motorcycle jumped so high that he rode into a cloud. The moisture in the cloud fouled his carburetor and he crashed to the ground.

The spirit of the ghost rider can sometimes be invoked. Everyone holds on to the edge of the parachute with both hands. One player raises his arms and quickly brings them down again. The player to his right follows, and then the next player in line, and so on. This movement creates a giant circular rolling wave.

A well-coordinated wave creates a jet of air that travels around and around underneath the parachute bringing forth the ghost rider. How fast can you get the ghost rider to rocket?

Lead-Ins Popcorn, Big Bang, Cat and Mouse, Shark, Rabbit and Hound.

Developmental Skills Primary—cooperation, verbal contact, skillfulness and coordination; Secondary—adaptability, self-control, visual ability, reaction, strength.

Duration of Game A few minutes.

Appropriate Ages Players younger than 6 years old might find this a big challenge.

When to Play Middle.

Follow-Ups Ball Surfing, Alligator, Popovers, Parachute Volleyball, Dodge 'Em.

Variations "Ghost Rider" is the opposite of Ghost Rider. Everyone begins by holding the parachute at about shoulder height. Players send the ghost rider rolling along the edge of the chute by progressively dipping their section of the chute down, letting the ghost rider pass, and then returning the chute to shoulder height.

Teaching Tips   If you raise the chute too soon, the ghost rider stalls. The key to this game is waiting until the moment when the puff of air just reaches you and then raising your section of the parachute up high. Younger players may not see the timing that clearly. Try adding audible cues. Have each player say, "Now," as she or he raises the chute. Both the arm raise and the audible "Now" get passed on to the next player in line.

Gophers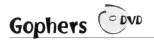

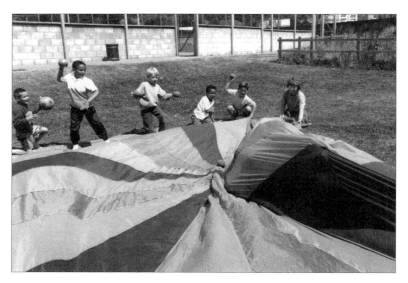

Spread the parachute out on the ground. All the players sit around the edge of the parachute holding on to it, except for a few gardeners who stand outside the parachute. Each gardener has a foam rubber ball. The gardeners ask players on one section of the parachute to become gophers and burrow under the parachute to the other side and back. While the gophers are crawling underneath the parachute, the gardeners try to hit them with a foam ball. If a gopher gets hit, he or she trades places with the gardener. The new gardeners ask a different pack of gophers to burrow under the chute for the next round. You might also allow those holding on to the parachute to throw a ball if it comes to them.

Lead-Ins Racing Heartbeat, Top of the Pops, Dodge 'Em, Wave Wall, Raceway.

Developmental Skills Primary— visual ability, reaction, crawling, throwing and catching, skillfulness and coordination, self-control, adaptability; Secondary—tactile contact, spontaneity.

Additional Equipment Three to five foam balls.

When to Play Middle.

Where to Play On a soft surface, excluding dirt.

Follow-Ups Sculpture, Centipede, Turnover, Treasure Hunt, Parachute Ride.

Variations   Revenge of the gophers! Give the balls to the gophers, with a chance to get back at the gardeners. Gardeners step up to hold the chute about chest high and are allowed to make waves to protect themselves. Gophers must stay under the center of the parachute in order to throw the ball at a gardener. Some of the gophers are needed outside of the parachute to retrieve errant balls. Be sure to rotate the inside gophers with the outside gophers so that everyone has the opportunity to both throw and retrieve the balls. Also, don't forget to switch so that the gardeners have a chance to be gophers.

Teaching Tips   In the excitement of the game, some gophers may not feel a small, light foam ball hitting them. Some gophers may even deny that they were hit. You can easily modify the game so that all gophers last for only one round, whether they were hit or not.

Heartbeat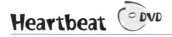

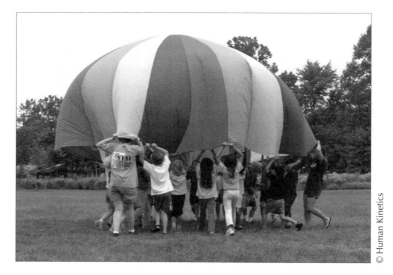

© Human Kinetics

Here's how to create a nice, steady heartbeat. Everyone gets into a steady rhythm by making a mushroom, walking in a step or two, and then walking back out as the parachute falls. When the blood has left the parachute, the players all lift up the chute and step in again to keep the heartbeat going.

Lead-Ins   Mushroom, Giant Mushroom, Wave Machine, Popcorn.

Developmental Skills   Primary—cooperation, adaptability, strength; Secondary—visual ability.

When to Play   Beginning.

Where to Play   Requires a tall ceiling if playing indoors.

Follow-Ups   Racing Heartbeat, Igloo, Floating Mushroom, other mushroom games.

Variations   Ask your players, "What would it look like if the parachute were to model the heart of a jogger? A sprinter? Someone who is sleeping?"

Teaching Tips   This is a nice, gentle game that lets first-time players discover the magic of a parachute. Make sure that all players have a comfortable grip around the edge, with a couple of rolls of parachute tucked under their fingers.

It's in the Bag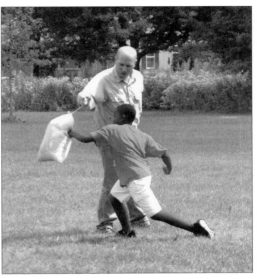

Don't think that you are necessarily through playing with the parachute just because it is all rolled up in the stuff bag. One time we were playing with a group of very aggressive kids. The play session was officially over, but the players were not ready to stop playing. One of them expressed his frustration by running up and kicking the duffel bag that was holding the parachute.

Not only was it a good release for him, but it also looked like fun. The others wanted to try it. It didn't hurt the duffel bag or the parachute, so we said, "Why not?" A line quickly formed, and we took turns loosely holding the bag while all the kids had a chance to run up and kick it. Everyone had a turn, we all felt better, and we were ready to get on with the next activity.

Instead of a line, you can keep the kids on their toes by having them form a large circle around you and the duffel bag. All the players around the circle must pay attention as the player who just kicked the bag calls out the name of the next player to enter the circle for a kick.

Lead-Ins Parachute Ride, Drag Race, Parachute Pass, Free Play, Group Balance.

Number of Players Fewer than 24. With more players than this, the thrill of being able to kick the bag does not quite match the tedium of waiting in line while the others have a turn.

Developmental Skills Primary—skillfulness and coordination; Secondary—cooperation, self-control, creativity, pantomime, visual ability, running, jumping.

Additional Equipment A durable bag to hold the parachute.

When to Play Ending.

Follow-Ups None—the parachute is in the bag.

Variations Instead of kicking the bag, it can also be punched. To make it a little more challenging, the trainer can raise or lower the bag as the kicker or puncher confronts the captive parachute.

You can also use the bagged parachute in any number of strength games. How far can one player toss the parachute? How about a mighty toss from four players, all working together? An entire Olympic decathlon could be played out, with the poor parachute substituting for the discus, javelin, shot put, long jumper, and whatnot.

Teaching Tips Check the condition of your parachute bag before playing this game. A sturdy bag, such as one made of canvas or another strong material, is best. Kids often have a lot of energy and pent-up aggression. We think it's better if this aggression is directed at the parachute rather than at each other or at you.

Liftoff

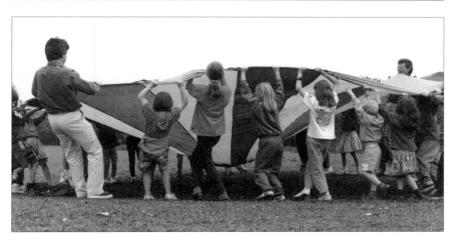

Does your waterbed have a leak? Here's how to make an air mattress. First, have everyone stretch the parachute out flat on the ground. Then a volunteer lies down in the middle. (If no one comes forward, guess who gets to volunteer!) Those holding the edge of the parachute should roll it up several times to prevent it from ripping. How far you roll the edge depends on how big the parachute is and how heavy the volunteer is: with a big parachute or a big person, you need to roll the edge up farther to make the diameter of the parachute smaller.

At a given signal, everyone lifts together, gently and slowly. (Remind all lifters to lift with their legs and keep their backs straight.) Sweet dreams for the person in the middle, at least for a minute. It's fun for the sleeper if those on the edge walk together in a circle. Don't forget to lower the sleeper gently so as not to cause a very rude awakening.

Safety Tips Especially with younger children, it is wise to have four or more adults spread around the perimeter of the parachute to ensure a soft landing for the sleeper.

Lead-Ins Group Balance, Sculpture, Wave Rolling, Centipede, Turnover.

Number of Players 12 or more.

Developmental Skills Primary—trust, strength, cooperation; Secondary—verbal contact, self-control, visual ability.

Appropriate Ages Players must be old enough and mature enough not to suddenly drop someone. We don't recommend Liftoff for players younger than 12 years of age.

When to Play   Middle.

Where to Play   Play this on a soft surface such as grass or mats—not on concrete.

Follow-Ups   Circular Tug, Circular Sit-Ups, Racing Heartbeat.

Variations   Divide the group into southern and northern hemispheres, as defined by the equator of the sleeper's body. Ask the inhabitants of the southern hemisphere to lower the chute slowly and gently to see if they can get the person in the middle to roll down to Antarctica.

Teaching Tips   This game is much more fun when played over a soft surface, such as grass or a wrestling mat. Even over a soft surface, the most successful rounds of this game include the softest possible landings for the player being lifted. It also seems like a good time to repeat that parachutes are not designed to toss people. Not good for the chute or the person.

Missile Launch

10, 9, 8, 7, 6, 5, 4, 3, 2, 1 . . . Ignition . . . Liftoff! This bird has flown! To be honest, this game is not as dramatic as a real missile launch; but you do get to launch a missile, in a way. Four or five players, each one carrying a ball, go under the parachute. While members of mission control (those holding on to the outside of the parachute) make a mushroom, the missile launchers attempt to throw their balls through the hole in the center of the parachute. How many missiles can they launch in one mushroom? Be sure to give everyone a chance.

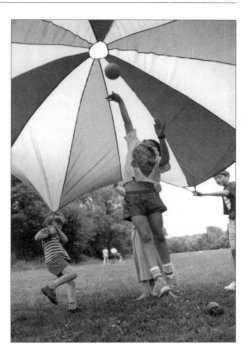

For a real challenge, ask the missile launchers to bounce their ball off the ground and through the hole.

Safety Tips   Use only soft foam balls.

Lead-Ins   Waves Overhead, Sculpture, Shark, any mushroom or popcorn games.

Developmental Skills   Primary—visual ability, throwing and catching, self-control, cooperation; Secondary—skillfulness and coordination, reaction, jumping.

Additional Equipment   Foam balls that fit through the hole in the center of the parachute.

Appropriate Ages   This may prove a great challenge for players younger than six.

When to Play   Middle.

Follow-Ups   Dodge 'Em, Treasure Hunt, Alligator, Centipede.

Variations   Hold an impromptu space race by dividing into two teams of competing rocket scientists. Teams take turns launching missiles from underneath the parachute. A team scores one point for each missile that escapes Earth's gravity and ascends to a successful orbit outside of the parachute.

It's easy to modify Missile Launch if your parachute does not have a hole in the center. Have the scientists stand around the outside of the parachute where they launch their missiles. The space vehicles orbit all the way over the top of the rising parachute and land on the other side. Launches must be really high or the missiles may end up crashing into the sun of the expanding parachute. You can also designate missile receivers who try to catch the falling spacecraft before they crash-land back to the Earth.

Teaching Tips   Smaller balls, with less mass and a smaller diameter, can escape Earth's gravity and make it through the hole in the center of the parachute much more easily than larger balls.

Parachute Basketball

Even an NBA super-star would find it hard to dunk in this game, because the basket is the hole in the middle of the parachute, high atop a mushroom.

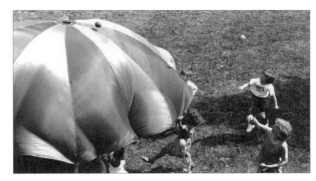

Four or five players, each with a ball, stand outside the edge of the parachute while the other players raise the parachute into a mushroom. Once the parachute is up, the shooters attempt to score baskets by throwing a ball through the hole. See how many balls get through the hole in one mushroom, or see how many mushrooms it takes to get one ball through. Naturally, you want to give everyone a chance, so alternate players after about five mushrooms. This may not get you on the all-star team, but it is a challenge, and it sure is fun.

Lead-Ins Missile Launch, Housekeeping, Big Bang, Popcorn, Top of the Pops.

Developmental Skills Primary—throwing and catching, self-control, visual ability, cooperation; Secondary—skillfulness and coordination, reaction, running, jumping.

Additional Equipment A foam ball for each basket shooter.

Appropriate Ages The under-6 age group may find this difficult.

When to Play Middle.

Follow-Ups Group Balance, Circular Sit-Ups, Flying Parachute.

Variations For a real challenge have people try to roll the foam balls up the side of the parachute and into the hole as in bowling, rather than shooting them into the hole as in basketball. The bowlers need to work closely with the mushroom makers in this game.

Teaching Tips The heavier the ball, the easier it will be to score a basket. A heavier ball will push the air out of the parachute faster. If the ball gets close enough, it just may collapse the chute enough to bring the hole within reach.

In our opinion, even though a heavier ball may make for a higher score, we don't recommend spending a lot of energy to find one. Sponge rubber balls work quite well for this activity. People have fun with this game, whether or not they score a lot of baskets.

Parachute Volleyball

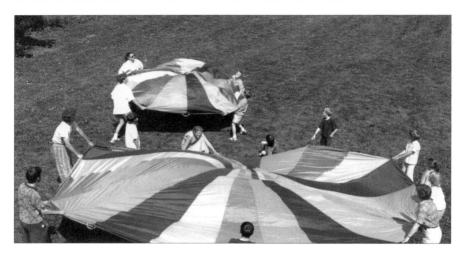

If you are lucky enough to have two small parachutes (both with a diameter of less than 12 feet, or 3.7 meters), you can use them together. For this game you also need a ball, the bigger the better. The goal is to play a version of volleyball. Each team has a parachute. The net is optional. The idea is to get the ball over to the other parachute. It takes a lot of teamwork not to send the ball flying out of control.

If you ever figure out a way to spike the ball, please let us know, and send a photo!

Lead-Ins   Interlocking Gears, any mushroom or popcorn games.

Number of Players   12 or more.

Developmental Skills   Primary—cooperation; Secondary—self-control, strength, problem solving, verbal contact, adaptability, visual ability.

Additional Equipment   A second parachute, a ball.

Appropriate Ages   May be too difficult for children under age 6.

When to Play   Middle.

Where to Play   Need enough room for least two fully opened parachutes.

Follow-Ups   Interlocking Gears, Big Bang, or any popcorn or mushroom games.

Variations   With two balls you could also have the teams play a modified version of the basketball game of HORSE. One team demonstrates a fancy move, or series of moves, with the ball and parachute. If the other team can't match the demonstration, it acquires a letter. In this game, as in the basketball version, the goal is to not end up with enough letters to spell "HORSE."

Teaching Tips   Teams should spread out their bigger and stronger players so that the lifting ability of the group is distributed equally. Also, inflatable beach balls are easy to lift but have a huge drag factor in the wind. Our experience has been that beach balls don't travel as far as foam balls.

Popovers

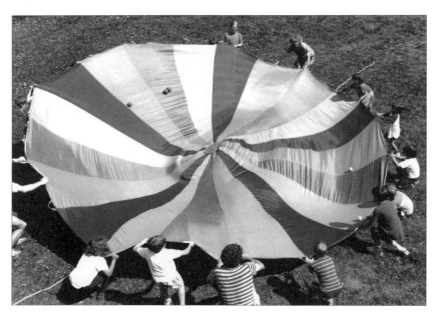

Divide the players into two teams facing each other across an imaginary line that is bisecting the parachute. Pull the parachute taut and place half the balls close to the edge on one team's side and the other half close to the edge on the opposite side. Each team tries to shake the parachute hard enough to make the balls pop over the heads of the other team.

One suggestion for making this challenge more interesting is to assign point values to different colored balls. Let's say all the yellow balls count as one point, and the red balls count as three. This should change the strategy a bit. Of course, once the game is over, who keeps track of the score?

Lead-Ins Wave Machine, Popcorn, Big Bang, any of the games with balls.

Developmental Skills Primary—cooperation, reaction; Secondary—verbal contact, self-control, spontaneity, adaptability, strength, endurance.

Additional Equipment Six balls, three of one color and three of another color.

Duration of Game Game may go very quickly but can be replayed several times.

Appropriate Ages Young children may by happy just to bounce the balls around.

When to Play   Middle.

Follow-Ups   Big Bang, Snake Tag, Gophers, Rabbit and Hound, other ball games.

Variations   Each team designates one or two free rovers. A free rover plays in the backfield, away from the parachute. Free rovers chase down all of the balls that fly off of the parachute and throw them back on, preferably on the other team's side. The round stops after a designated period (one to two minutes), and points are tallied by counting all of the balls the free rovers weren't able to return to the chute.

Teaching Tips   Make sure each side has an equal balance of big, strong players and small, not-as-strong ones.

Shark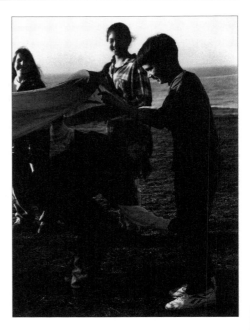

Let's go to the beach! Players hold the parachute about waist high and stretched taut. One player, the shark, goes underneath the parachute with a Frisbee. The shark holds the edge of the Frisbee against the underside of the parachute while circling underneath to make it look as if a shark fin is rising up out of the water. The other players can make small waves with the parachute to simulate the ocean and hum the soundtrack from the movie *Jaws:* "Dah-dum, dah-dum, dah-dum."

Watch out! The shark may decide to pretend-bite one of the players holding on to the edge of the parachute by grabbing a leg. This player then cries out, takes the Frisbee from the shark, and becomes the new shark. Warning: If there are enough Frisbees, a feeding frenzy might develop as more and more sharks enter the water!

Lead-Ins Wave Machine, World Record Merry-Go-Round, any mushroom games.

Developmental Skills Primary—tactile contact, spontaneity, pantomime, cooperation; Secondary—walking, verbal contact, adaptability, self-control, visual ability.

Additional Equipment Three to five Frisbees.

When to Play Middle.

Follow-Ups Turnover, Drag Race, Parachute Ride, It's in the Bag.

Variations In Vampire Shark the original shark never has to relinquish the Frisbee to create more sharks. Any human bitten by a shark mysteriously mutates into a shark to join the ever-growing school beneath the parachute. The round is over when there are no humans left, just some flotsam, jetsam, and a bunch of hungry sharks.

Teaching Tips No Frisbee? No problem! Just have players use their upturned hands for shark fins.

Treasure Hunt

Throw everything under the para- chute: balls, jump ropes, Frisbees, stale bread. Everything is fair game. Arrange all the players around the parachute and have them make a steady Heartbeat. On the upswing, point to one or more people to go under the para- chute, search for a particular treasure, 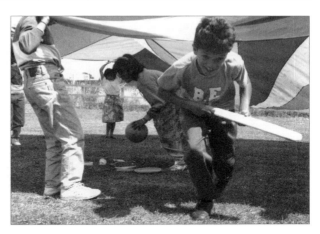 and bring it out. The Heartbeat provides an automatic time limit: If a seeker stays too long and gets touched by the parachute, she or he must rebury the treasure for the next round.

Safety Tips   Remind players to watch out for collisions when racing to col- lect treasure.

Lead-Ins   Heartbeat, Rabbit and Hound, Pony Express, Rocking Chair, Snake Tag.

Developmental Skills   Primary—self-control, visual ability, skillfulness and coordination, reaction; Secondary—problem solving, speed, running, coop- eration, verbal contact, adaptability.

Additional Equipment   Balls, jump ropes, Frisbees, stale bread, any avail- able small objects.

When to Play   Middle.

Follow-Ups   Racing Heartbeat, Popovers, Parachute Golf, Ostrich, Igloo.

Variations   In Buried Treasure players have the time of one heartbeat to carry treasure from outside of the parachute and leave it buried underneath.

Teaching Tips   There should be a maximum of three treasure hunters under the chute at any given time. More than that and the brave buccaneers risk being keelhauled. Although we aren't exactly sure what that means, we don't want to find out.

Wave Machine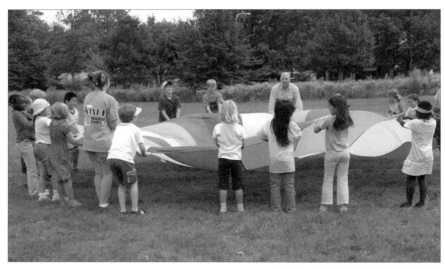

The easiest parachute game and the one everyone plays without any prompting is Wave Machine. Simply spread out the parachute, grab an edge, and begin to shake. Tiny ripples will soon turn into frothy waves.

Lead-In   Free Play.

Developmental Skills   Primary—strength, endurance; Secondary—cooperation, self-control.

When to Play   Beginning.

Follow-Ups   Popcorn games or a low-activity game to give players a rest.

Variations   Have groups of three or four players, who are concentrated together along one arc of the parachute, take turns sending a large wave directly across to the players on the opposite shore.

Teaching Tips   This is another game that is an excellent introduction to the parachute. You may want to glance around and see that everyone has a comfortable grip on the edge of the parachute.

Waves Overhead

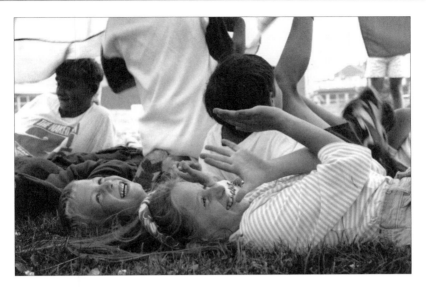

Would the group like to give a great gift to a couple of players? Send three to five scuba divers in to lie down under the parachute while the rest of the players vigorously shake the parachute. This makes strong waves over the divers. It's a great way to cool off on a hot day.

Lead-Ins   Heartbeat, Racing Heartbeat, Dodge 'Em, Jellyfish Jaunt, Raceway.

Developmental Skills   Primary—strength, endurance; Secondary—cooperation, self-control, tactile contact.

When to Play   Middle.

Follow-Ups   Centipede, Cop and Robber, Flying Parachute, Cat and Mouse.

Variations   Players who are underneath the parachute must remain on their backs. Toss some foam balls on top of the chute. You have just created a version of keep-away. Players around the parachute make waves to keep the balls away from the players who are underneath.

Teaching Tips   Scuba divers don't just have to lie passively underneath the chute. They can choose to kneel, crawl, or swim around in any manner they like, as long as they don't endanger other aquatic life.

High-Activity
Parachute Games

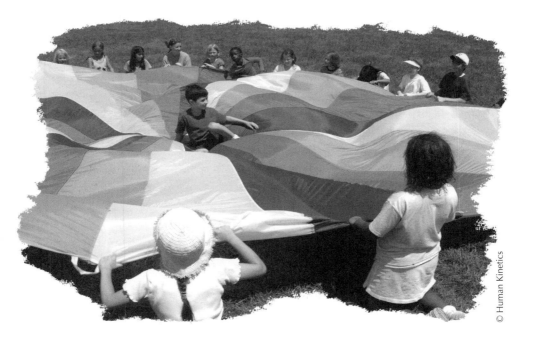

© Human Kinetics

Name	Page number	When to play	Included on DVD
Cat and Mouse	123	Middle	⊙
Flying Parachute	125	Middle	
Housekeeping	126	Middle	
I Dare Ya	127	Middle	
Jell-O	129	Middle	⊙
Jellyfish Jaunt	130	Middle	
Merry-Go-Round	132	Middle	⊙
Pony Express	134	Middle	
Popcorn	136	Beginning	⊙
Raceway	137	Middle	
Racing Heartbeat	138	Middle	⊙
Snake Tag	140	Middle	⊙
Top of the Pops	141	Middle	
Wave Rolling	142	Middle	
World Record Merry-Go-Round	143	Middle	⊙

Playing with a parachute is a pretty exciting experience, and here are 15 of the most exciting high-activity games. If attention is waning, try one of these!

Cat and Mouse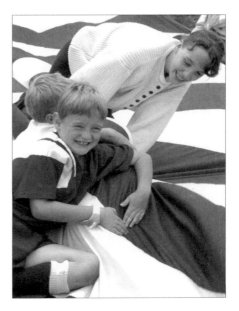

Cats chase mice. To protect themselves, the mice in this game hide under the parachute. Everyone else holds the parachute loosely at about waist level. Whoever has a birthday closest to June 9 (or any date you prefer) gets to be under the parachute as the mouse. The player wearing the most yellow gets on top of the parachute as the cat.

The cat closes its eyes while everyone begins making small waves to help hide the mouse. The mouse stays low and scurries underneath the parachute to avoid the cat. The cat, which is on all four paws, opens its eyes and tries to catch the mouse underneath all the waves. Usually the cat has a time limit with everyone counting out loud in unison down from 20 or some other appropriate number. Then for the next round, the cat and mouse pick replacements from the group of players who have not yet been chosen to play.

Depending on the size (i.e., age) and number of your players, you might want to experiment with different numbers of cats and mice. Here are two different strategies: Players can use the parachute either to help the mouse escape from the cat or to reveal the mouse to the cat by holding the parachute down momentarily. Please play fairly with this tip.

Safety Tips   Avoid playing on concrete or blacktop. Cats and mice may get scrapes and bruises, and the hard surface may tear the parachute.

Lead-Ins   Racing Heartbeat, Free Play, most low- or moderate-activity games.

Developmental Skills   Primary—cooperation, tactile contact, visual ability, reaction, leaning, crawling; Secondary—verbal contact, self-control, spontaneity, strength, endurance.

Duration of Game   This game could go on until everyone gets a turn being a cat or mouse.

When to Play   Middle.

Where to Play   Best played on a soft surface such as mats. It can also be played on grass, if you don't mind grass stains on everyone's clothing and the parachute.

Follow-Ups   Any low- or moderate-activity game, such as Circular Sit-Ups.

Variations   Place an object such as an inflated inner tube on top of the center of the parachute. This will weigh down the center and create an open ring between the center and outside of the parachute for the cat to chase the mouse.

Teaching Tips   The donut variation is especially useful if the cat is having a difficult time finding the mouse.

Flying Parachute

Have everyone gather on the edge of one half of the parachute and hold the edge with one hand. Everyone takes off running in the same direction. This gives the impression of trying to launch a giant wounded kite.

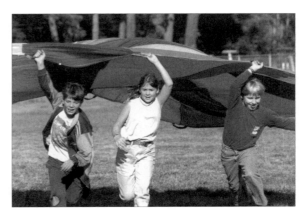

Safety Tips Remind players to watch where they're going! Sometimes they get so caught up in the excitement that they forget to watch for holes, water sprinklers, and other low-altitude hazards.

Lead-Ins Group Balance, Igloo, Blow Up, Turnover, Ostrich, Big Bang.

Number of Players 24 or fewer.

Developmental Skills Primary—cooperation, reaction, endurance, running; Secondary—verbal contact, adaptability, self-control, visual ability, strength.

When to Play Middle.

Where to Play Find a place that has enough space to allow for a good run.

Follow-Ups Liftoff, Parachute Pass, Who's Peeking?, Missile Launch, Free Play.

Variations Divide the players into two groups. Members of one group lie down on their backs, head to toe, in a single line. Players in the other group hold both sides of the chute, with a nice, large gap between the two lines of players on either side of the chute. The idea is to sail the parachute directly over the people who are lying down. A colorful, flapping parachute seen up close is quite a sight.

Teaching Tips A great practical joke to play on bystanders is to ask one or two players to chase the flying parachute yelling, "Bring back my handkerchief!"

Housekeeping

A team of three or four players stands a bit away from the parachute. This is the neatness team. Their job is to make sure that all the balls stay on the parachute. Meanwhile, the messy team, holding the parachute, is trying to shake all the balls off the parachute. At the end of 30 seconds or so, everyone stops to tally up how many balls are on the parachute and how many are off. Select a new neatness team and repeat until everyone has had a turn to be neat.

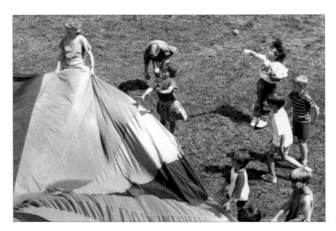

Lead-Ins   Wave Machine, Popcorn, Snake Tag, Ostrich, or any less active game.

Developmental Skills   Primary—cooperation, adaptability, self-control, visual ability, strength, throwing and catching; Secondary—problem solving, verbal contact, spontaneity, endurance, running.

Additional Equipment   At least more foam balls than players on the neatness team.

When to Play   Middle.

Follow-Ups   Parachute Basketball, Pony Express, Waves Overhead, Cat and Mouse.

Variations   Instead of holding rounds to have players change roles, you can institute the tap exchange. After a player from the neat team cleans up a mess by throwing a ball back on the parachute, she or he taps one of the messy players along the edge of the chute. After the tap, both players switch positions.

Teaching Tips   Although we suggest that each round should last about 30 seconds, the actual amount of time for a round depends on the group. Check to see that your players' arms aren't getting tired. A great way to tell if peoples' arms are tired is to be a fellow player. If your arms are tired, so are the arms of your players.

I Dare Ya

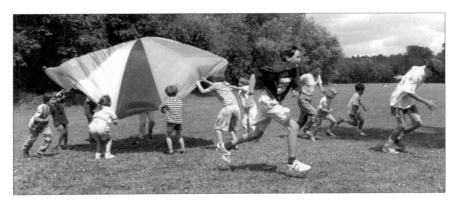

Two teams—composed of every other person—are evenly spread out around the parachute. Both teams make steady heartbeats together. The teams take turns challenging each other to complete some goal before a set number of heartbeat pulses. The challenge can be fulfilled underneath, around, or completely away from the parachute.

For example, one dare might be for each team member to touch his or her toes in one pulse. Easy. A different challenge could be for everyone to touch a door and come back to the parachute in two pulses.

A dare does not have to involve the entire team. One representative of the team might be challenged to do 10 push-ups in two pulses. Or the goal could require that the entire team work together, perhaps forming a line long enough to have someone touch a tree while the other end holds on to the parachute in three heartbeats.

Be careful not to make too tough of a challenge. The challenged team has the option to contest the dare. This means that the challenging team must attempt to perform its own feat.

Safety Tips   No dare should be truly dangerous.

Lead-Ins   Heartbeat, any mushroom game, any low- or moderate-activity game.

Developmental Skills   Primary—reaction, endurance, self-control; Secondary—cooperation, verbal contact, tactile contact, creativity, visual ability, skillfulness and coordination, running, hopping, problem solving, adaptability, spontaneity.

When to Play   Middle.

Where to Play   Best to have some space around the parachute for more dare possibilities.

Follow-Ups   Treasure Hunt, Turnover, or any less active game.

Variations   If a group accepts and fails to meet a challenge, the original challengers have the option to win further glory by meeting their own challenge.

Teaching Tips   Be prepared to offer some preliminary challenges to give players some ideas.

Jell-O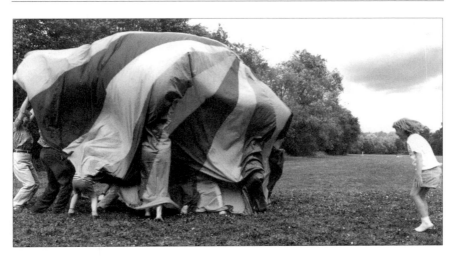

Everyone crawls underneath the parachute, except for a couple of cooks who remain outside. These cooks want to make People Jell-O. They ask the ingredients (players) to move or raise certain body parts to make forms under the parachute. For instance, a cook might call out, "Three jumping jacks" or "Lie on your back and raise your left leg straight up." If a cook chooses to taste the creation, he or she changes places with someone under the parachute.

Lead-Ins   Racing Heartbeat, Sculpture, Cop and Robber, Floating Mushroom, Shark.

Developmental Skills   Primary—visual ability, crawling; Secondary—cooperation, verbal contact, tactile contact, creativity, pantomime, skillfulness and coordination, jumping, hopping.

When to Play   Middle.

Follow-Ups   Climb the Mountain, Gophers, Parachute Basketball, Wave Rolling.

Variations   Through instantaneous evolution Jell-O sometimes develops a mind of its own. In this version the Jell-O has free will and can choose to determine its own fate. The cooks on the outside of the parachute become guessers, trying to figure out what the heck the Jell-O is doing.

Teaching Tips   Cooks may be too shy or overwhelmed to suggest activities for the Jell-O. If the cooks have a hard time coming up with ideas, we have found it is helpful to ask specific questions to help prompt ideas. "What should the Jell-O do with its feet?" "Should the Jell-O bend its collective waist or keep it straight?"

Jellyfish Jaunt

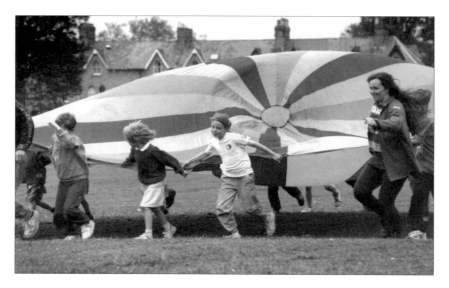

One day a group of players asked if they could take a run with the parachute. Well, why not? Everyone gathered around the parachute and took off. It looked as if the world's largest multicolored jellyfish was let loose in the park. Could this be the subject for the next Stephen King novel?

Safety Tips   Players need to watch for anyone who happens to fall. In fact, the jellyfish should avoid passing too closely to or running over any object because the following side might not see the object and could get into a real jam! As always when running, be aware of holes, sprinkler heads, and so on.

Lead-Ins   Sculpture, Turnover, Inflating the Parachute, any low-activity games.

Number of Players   12 or more.

Developmental Skills   Primary—endurance, running; Secondary—cooperation, verbal contact, adaptability, spontaneity, self-control, visual ability.

When to Play   Middle.

Where to Play   Give yourself enough space for a decent run.

Follow-Ups   Free Play, Ostrich, Who's Peeking?, Cover Up, any low-activity games.

Variations   First, have the jellyfish slow down to a slow jog. Can the back of the jellyfish overtake the front of the jellyfish, with everyone continuing to hold on to the chute? This becomes a moveable version of Over Under (page 69). Two players at the front of the jellyfish slide away from each other to make a gate for the back of the jellyfish to pass through. A jaunting jellyfish that turns itself inside out should be proud. You are demonstrating precision that would make a marching band proud.

Teaching Tips   This game can be tiring. We have had energetic groups that didn't notice how tiring this game can be nearly as quickly as we did. As a change of pace, and to catch your breath, suggest that the jellyfish hop, skip, jump, or gallop for a spell. You can also slow things down by asking the players to have the parachute undulate like a real jellyfish as it goes for a jaunt.

Merry-Go-Round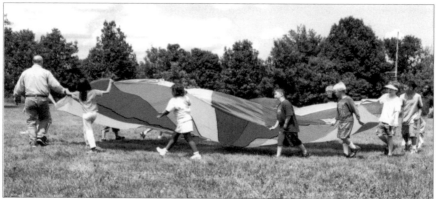

This game brings back the spirit of the old carousels. Everyone grabs an edge of the parachute with one hand and begins walking in a giant circle. To really get into the mood, you can start bobbing up and down as you walk, just like the wooden horses.

Got the idea? Have everyone run a lap, and then have them jump on both feet for a lap. How about hopping on one foot? Or alternate five hops on the left foot with five on the right. Can you all skip together while holding the parachute? How about a gallop? After a while, switch directions.

Lead-Ins   Flying Parachute, Jellyfish Jaunt, any lower-activity game.

Developmental Skills   Primary—walking, jumping, hopping; Secondary—cooperation, skillfulness and coordination, endurance, verbal contact, adaptability, self-control, balancing.

When to Play   Middle.

Follow-Ups   World Record Merry-Go-Round, any lower-activity game.

Variations   Players pair up and stand next to each other, facing the same direction. The pairs form two circles radiating out from the parachute, creating an inside and an outside circle. The inside half of each pair holds on to the chute with her or his left hand. The right hand of the insider holds the left hand of the outsider. The outsider's right hand is free. As the pairs walk around the merry-go-round, they alternate bobbing up and down, just like an old-time carousel.

In Detective, two or three players stand outside the circle, briefly closing their eyes or looking in the other direction while the group chooses a leader. After a leader is chosen, the group begins a round of Merry-Go-Round, silently following the lead of the one who was chosen. If the leader starts hopping, everyone hops around the Merry-Go-Round; when the leader begins walking, everyone imitates with walking. All of the players try to switch as quickly as possible to mask the identity of the secret leader. The detectives' job is to determine the identity of the leader.

Teaching Tips   Merry-Go-Round is another excellent introduction to playing with a parachute. At the same time, the activity consists of nothing more than a group of people walking around in a circle. Watch the interest level of the group, and be ready to move to another game when their interest begins to wane.

Pony Express

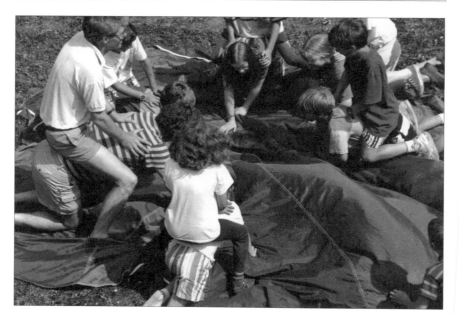

Part of the history of the West in the United States is the courageous Pony Express riders that galloped across treacherous terrain to deliver mail. The journey was too long and arduous for one rider to complete, so a group of riders each took on one smaller section, passing the mail forward in a type of long-distance relay race.

We can re-create the varied landscape of the Old West and the hurried rush to deliver the mail in this game. Players pair up: One person goes under the parachute while the teammate stands outside. The player underneath sits or crouches under the parachute facing out and is the first Pony Express rider. The outside player faces in, holds on to the parachute, and is the second rider. All the second riders lift the parachute up. This releases the first riders, who crawl between their partner's legs and run around the parachute. While the riders are running, the second riders make a mushroom and get down on all fours, bringing the parachute with them.

When the first riders reach their destination, their partners, they symbolically hand off the mail package by tagging the second rider. The second riders must cross the giant mountain looming before them by crawling across the parachute and running around the outside back to the first rider.

Pony Express is similar to Climb the Mountain, with a bit more activity before the climbing begins.

Safety Tips The same safety tips from Climb the Montain apply to Pony Express; remind the players to be aware of others as they cross over the mountain.

It's a good idea to pair players of similar size so that one doesn't get squished. Remind riders that the saddle is back on the pony's hips, not on their poor pony's back.

Lead-Ins Cat and Mouse, Climb the Mountain, Igloo, Rocking Chair, Centipede.

Developmental Skills Primary—tactile contact, skillfulness and coordination, leaning, crawling; Secondary—cooperation, verbal contact, self-control, visual ability, reaction, balancing.

When to Play Middle.

Where to Play A soft surface is best.

Follow-Ups Treasure Hunt, Waves Overhead, Cop and Robber, Gophers, Shark.

Variations You can have riders pass through a giant tunnel by having them crawl underneath the parachute instead of over it.

Teaching Tips Pony Express is one of the more complicated games in this book. Be prepared for some fun confusion as the Pony Express riders tag or forget to tag their partners before crossing the Continental Divide. It will help some players better understand their roles if you call, "Freeze!" in between the three stages. While the players are frozen, you can remind them what they should do for the next stage.

Popcorn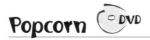

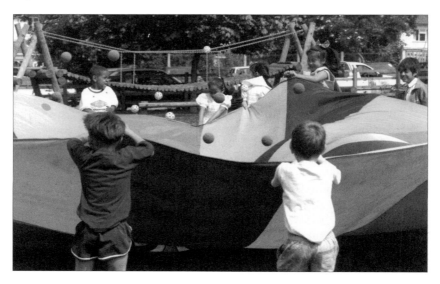

If you have lots of soft balls, you can make a giant popcorn machine. Just throw the light, spongy balls onto the parachute. People will get the idea.

Activity Level   Moderate to high.

Lead-Ins   Wave Machine, Shark, Mushroom, and low-activity games.

Developmental Skills   Primary—endurance; Secondary—self-control, spontaneity, visual ability, reaction, strength, throwing and catching.

Additional Equipment   At least three (or as many as you have) foam balls or other soft, bouncy objects.

When to Play   Beginning.

Follow-Ups   Mushroom, Jellyfish Jaunt, any moderate- or low-activity game.

Variations   What would it like look if everyone tried to cook up a batch of risotto, rather than pop popcorn? Risotto needs to be stirred gently and constantly, or it will stick to the sides. Without making any waves, everyone needs to swish the parachute around and around to keep all of the balls rolling around on top of the chute.

Teaching Tips   If you are ever stuck for an idea, just toss some foam balls on the chute and let folks have fun. This gives you an excellent opportunity to consult your list of games for the next idea.

Raceway

This is good training for rush-hour traffic. Everyone holds on to the parachute and walks in a circle as in Merry-Go-Round. The leader calls out different instructions and explains who is to do what. For example, all left-handers might be asked to pass two drivers in front of them. The left-handed players would then let go of the parachute and try to pass the two right-handed people in front of them who are still holding on to the parachute. The object of the game is to get to the head of the circle, just like driving on the raceway.

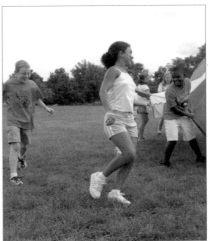
© Human Kinetics

For a real workout, have players jog while they are holding the parachute. For more variety, have players switch directions.

Safety Tips   Choose an area free from obstacles so that the commuters can run safely.

Lead-Ins   Cover Up, Free Play, Circular Tug, Swooping Cloud, mushroom games.

Developmental Skills   Primary—endurance, running; Secondary—adaptability, self-control, visual ability, verbal contact.

When to Play   Middle.

Follow-Ups   Ghost Rider, Group Balance, Parachute Pass, Turnover, Drag Race.

Variations   Have you ever wanted to avoid a traffic jam by taking a shortcut? That's easy to accomplish in Raceway. Instead of using the outside lane, specified drivers create a shortcut by crossing directly under the chute. Their goal is to time the shortcut in such a way that they can tuck back into traffic on the edge of the parachute in their customary position. Although it turns out that taking shortcuts doesn't actually result in any progress in the line, it sure is fun.

Teaching Tips   We have found that lots of groups get into the audible aspect of Raceway. Is it a universal fascination with cars, trucks, and motorcycles that causes the players to rev up their engines with various lip, tongue, and throat sounds? Whatever the reason, it seems to add to the enjoyment of the game.

Racing Heartbeat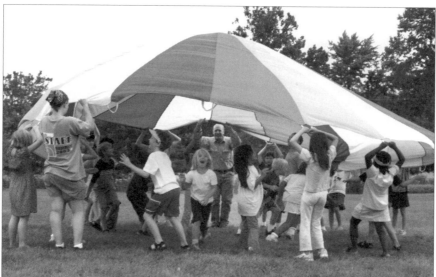

© Human Kinetics

Once you establish the heartbeat, you can have people cross under the parachute while it is in the air. Be careful! Everyone will want to run under the parachute at the same time. To prevent total pandemonium, you should take time to explain the activity first, clarify that everyone will get a chance to cross under, and state that you will announce specific categories describing who should cross.

For instance, as the parachute is going up, ask people who are wearing certain types or colors of clothes to cross under the parachute. Or you can select players by their birth month. You can also choose players according to their favorite flavor of ice cream: strawberry, chocolate, or vanilla. Or you could find out who has a cat by seeing who crosses under when you call out, "All those with cats!" Or you can see who prefers history to mathematics. For a big surprise call out any all-inclusive category, such as all those born between January 1 and December 31.

Safety Tips Be sure to remind players to watch out for others as they run underneath the parachute. (Everyone tends to converge in the middle.) Although contact with other players is fine, we don't want to have any high-speed, jarring collisions between players.

Warning Sometimes people mistakenly think the object of the game is to bring the parachute down quickly on one of the runners. Unfortunately, this strategy can lower the edge of the parachute down to the same level as the neck of someone who is running fairly fast; this, of course, can be rather dangerous. It is important to stress to the players that the heartbeat must maintain a steady speed.

Lead-Ins   Heartbeat, Mushroom, Giant Mushroom, low-activity games.

Developmental Skills   Primary—cooperation, trust, adaptability, visual ability, strength; Secondary—verbal contact, tactile contact, self-control, creativity, running.

When to Play   Middle.

Follow-Ups   Floating Parachute, Over Under, Flying Parachute, low-activity games.

Variations   Don't forget to vary the means of locomotion, as well as the category. While people born in April may run across, those born in September hop across, or whatever the caller decides.

Teaching Tips   This is a great opportunity to have even the shy players get used to being callers. The position of caller can rotate along the perimeter of the parachute. This can also lead to some confusion and fun. While the position of caller ticks along the perimeter, one stop at a time, the players are changing their positions in a random manner. Players are sometimes surprised to arrive at a new spot on the parachute and realize that they must quickly call out a new category.

Snake Tag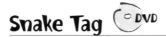

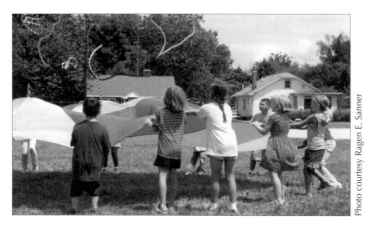

Photo courtesy Ragen E. Sanner

Throw a bunch of short ropes on the parachute. Divide the parachute down the middle into two opposing teams. The object is to shake the parachute so vigorously that a snake bites someone on the other team. Watch out that you don't get bitten yourself!

You may find that young children simply enjoy making the ropes bounce.

Safety Tips   Jump ropes work well only if they don't have heavy, dangerous handles.

Activity Level   Moderate to high.

Lead-Ins   Wave Machine, Popcorn, Big Bang, Popovers, any of the games with balls.

Developmental Skills   Primary—strength; Secondary—adaptability, self-control, visual ability, reaction, endurance.

Additional Equipment   Ropes that measure four to six feet (1.2 to 1.8 meters) in length.

When to Play   Middle.

Follow-Ups   A somewhat lower-activity game, such as Ostrich or Igloo.

Variations   Instead of dividing the group into two teams, have everyone work together to try to get the snakes to slither down the hole in the center of the parachute.

Teaching Tips   Although it is tempting, resist the urge to ask the players to try to shake the parachute deftly enough to tie the snakes up in knots. Even the most sophisticated playgroups find this too challenging.

Top of the Pops

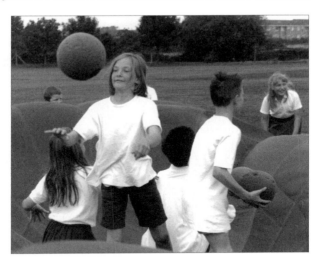

One group of players spontaneously started to play this game. We liked it, so we are including it here. The game is set up like Popcorn but has people added on top of the parachute. The three or four people who are on the parachute try to throw the bouncing balls off. Popcorn poppers, those who are around the edge of the parachute, holding it and shaking it, try to keep the popcorn in the popper. In other words, they retrieve the balls and toss them back onto the parachute. Just for fun, you can yell, "Freeze!" after playing for a minute or two and see how many balls of popcorn are on the parachute and how many are off the parachute.

Safety Tips   It's best not to use hard or even inflated balls. Somebody inevitably ends up getting whacked in the head.

Lead-Ins   Popcorn, Big Bang, Parachute Volleyball, any less active game.

Developmental Skills   Primary—throwing and catching, self-control, visual ability, reaction, strength, crawling; Secondary—tactile contact, endurance, spontaneity, skillfulness and coordination.

Additional Equipment   Four or five foam balls (any other kind might roll away too far).

When to Play   Middle.

Follow-Ups   Snake Tag, popcorn games, any less active game.

Variations   Make it more challenging for the people on top of the chute by imposing soccer-style rules. These folks aren't allowed to touch the balls with their hands; only kicks and headers are legal.

Teaching Tips   This high-energy game can be both fun and tiring. A good way to see how the popcorn poppers are doing is to notice the average height of the balls. As poppers get tired, the popcorn starts to settle down into the bottom of the pan.

Wave Rolling

After people see the parachute as a Wave Machine, many want to get on top. So let them. For the best all-around experience, limit the number of players on the parachute to five. Everyone around the edge gets to make waves. With 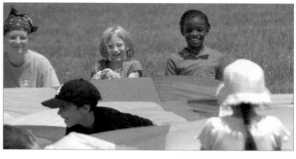 too many on the parachute or too few wave makers, it looks as though you are sailing through the doldrums.

Once the storm begins, you will find out how seaworthy people are as they crawl and roll around on the waves.

Safety Tips   Ask those on the waves to get on their hands and knees. Waves are difficult to walk on without falling, especially on a hard surface. You may also want players on the waves to remove their shoes for each other's and the parachute's safety.

Activity Level   Moderate to high.

Lead-Ins   Wave Machine, Rabbit and Hound, Popcorn, Parachute Golf.

Developmental Skills   Primary—crawling, endurance, strength, trust, adaptability; Secondary—self-control, creativity, tactile contact, visual ability, problem solving, spontaneity.

When to Play   Middle.

Where to Play   Best played on a soft surface such as grass, carpeting, or mats.

Follow-Ups   Top of the Pops, Snake Tag, Popovers, Pony Express, Cat and Mouse.

Variations   Toss a couple of foam balls into the ocean. Wave rollers start in the middle, adrift at sea, and try to swim to shore without being touched by any of the ocean foam. Wave makers on the edge of the chute start to make waves. Each roller, after making it safely to shore, picks a new roller for the next round.

Teaching Tips   You will quickly find out that it is easier for the group to make waves if the players on top of the parachute move about near the center rather than at the edge of the chute.

World Record Merry-Go-Round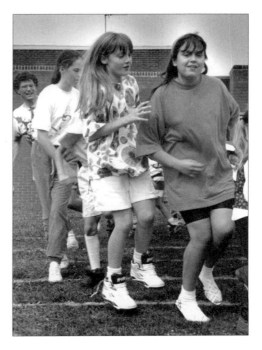

Set a Frisbee or some other marker on the ground outside but near the parachute, and you can play a competitive version of Merry-Go-Round. What is interesting is that the group ends up competing against itself.

Use a stopwatch to time how long it takes the players to make one complete revolution clockwise, stop, and then return to the same starting position by going counterclockwise. Now, can we beat that record?

Safety Tips   Make sure that players watch out for little ones in a mixed-age group. Sometimes they fall and risk getting trodden on, or they fall while holding on to the parachute, in which case they may get dragged.

Lead-Ins   Merry-Go-Round, Cover Up, Group Balance, Parachute, Blow Up, Ostrich, Igloo.

Developmental Skills   Primary—running, jumping, hopping; Secondary—cooperation, endurance, verbal contact, adaptability, self-control, skillfulness and coordination, reaction, balancing.

When to Play   Middle.

Follow-Ups   Parachute Pass, Who's Peeking?, Drag Race, any lower-activity game.

Variations   Let's continue with the idea of combining the parachute with a watch. Imagine that the parachute is a giant clock. All of the players hold on to the edge of the parachute and represent the tips of hour hands along the watch. Of course, since there are only 12 hours on a clock face, some of the players may represent minutes between the hours.

Place a Frisbee on the ground about 6 feet (1.8 meters) away from one of the players. The Frisbee designates the 12 o'clock position. The player who is closest to the Frisbee is at 12 o'clock. The player farthest away on the other side of the parachute is at 6 o'clock.

When all of the players have become familiar with their positions on the clock face, it is time for the game to begin. Announce that four hours have passed. Everyone must quickly move the parachute to represent the new time. The player who was directly in front of the Frisbee should now be at the four o'clock position. The player who was at eight o'clock should end up standing nearest the Frisbee.

The person standing nearest the Frisbee announces how many hours have elapsed for the next round. Don't forget: In this game time flows both forward and backward. It's perfectly appropriate to ask the clock to show how it looked seven hours ago.

If your group is very adept at telling time, you can designate one player to let go of the parachute, step back a couple of feet from the chute, and represent the minute hand. Now everyone is free to call out both how many hours and how many minutes have changed since the players last looked at the clock.

Teaching Tips If you have a group of players who aren't comfortable telling time, you can vary the game by having them count off different numbers of steps as they march around the circle in a clockwise or counterclockwise direction. If the entire group takes four giant steps in one direction, have them find out how many tiny steps it will take to get back to the original location.

On page 16 we advised that you hold a practice round when introducing a new game. Don't mention "practice round" to any of the players, and you can use the secret concept of an undisclosed practice round to guarantee success with World Record Merry-Go-Round.

It turns out that every single group we have ever played with finds it quite easy to break its own record. The first time a group tries an activity, any activity, the attempt is, at best, tentative. Many players will not be sure if they understand what they are supposed to do, so they will hold back a bit to check and see that they aren't doing anything wrong.

Even with a thorough understanding of what is expected, the first attempt of almost any physical activity has a large amount of uncertainty attached to it. "Is this the best way to go around quickly in a circle?"

Having seen how the game is played, after even one trial run (the unspoken "practice round"), any group will be ready, willing, and able to break its previous record, thus shattering the world record for this game.

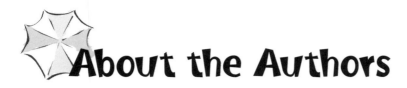

About the Authors

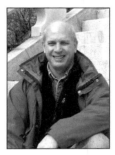

Todd Strong worked as lead trainer for the New Games Foundation, a nonprofit organization that teaches personal and professional development by bringing people closer together through play. In this position, he traveled throughout the United States conducting workshops, during which he was able to collect and try out parachute games in many settings and with different groups. As the foundation's program director, he planned and promoted New Games and New Games workshops worldwide.

A past chairman and director and current active member of the International Jugglers' Association, Todd has authored many books on juggling, including *The Devil Stick Book, The Dice Stacking Book, The Diabolo Book,* and *Diabolo for Advanced Players.* He taught juggling as a Jonglierlehrer in Germany and as a *professeur de jonglerie* at the national circus school of France, in addition to many short courses and workshops throughout North America and Europe.

Todd's education seems to be on a northward drift. He earned a bachelor's degree in recreation from California State University at Hayward, a master's in experiential education from Mankato State University in Minnesota, and a master's in adult education from the University of British Columbia in Canada.

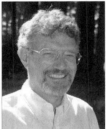

Dale N. LeFevre, a native of Wisconsin, started working in San Francisco as a volunteer with the nonprofit New Games Foundation in 1975. By the start of 1976 he was office manager and associate director. In 1977 he formed his own project, which took New Games into schools. In 1979 he left the United States for eight years to promote New Games around the world, presenting workshops in every major European country plus South Africa, Israel, India, Japan, Australia, and New Zealand.

LeFevre's previous publications include *New Games for the Whole Family* (eventually published in five languages and due to be reprinted under a new title) and *Parachute Games.* He has also produced or coproduced the *New Games CD-ROM* and several videos, including *The New Games Video, New Games From Around the World, Rainy Day Games, Sunny Day Games, New Soccer (For Fun and Skills), Cooperative Group Games,* and *Skill Games.* His latest production is *The New Parachute Games Video,* which was just made into *The New Parachute Games DVD.*

On the immediate horizon are two more DVDs, *Cooperative Games DVD* and *The New Games DVD.* LeFevre has founded a new company, Playworks, which works with businesses to use New Games to improve communication, build stronger teams, and reduce stress.

LeFevre holds a master's degree in education from New York University and a bachelor's degree in business from Valparaiso University. In his free time he enjoys gardening, hiking, biking, and camping. As of 2006, he lives in Sheffield, England.

*You'll find
other outstanding
physical activity resources at*

www.HumanKinetics.com

In the U.S. call

1-800-747-4457

Australia.............................. 08 8372 0999
Canada 1-800-465-7301
Europe...................... +44 (0) 113 255 5665
New Zealand.................. 0064 9 448 1207